the
MEMORY
book

the
MEMORY
book

Judith Wiles & Janet Wiles

ABC
Books

Published by ABC Books for the
AUSTRALIAN BROADCASTING CORPORATION
GPO Box 9994 Sydney NSW 2001

Copyright © Judith Wiles and Janet Wiles 2003

First published 2003
Reprinted December 2003
Reprinted April 2004
Reprinted August 2004
Reprinted September 2006

National Library of Australia
Cataloguing-in-Publication entry:

Wiles, Judith.
The memory book: everyday habits for a healthy memory.

Includes index.
ISBN 0 7333 1169 5.
ISBN 978 0 7333 1169 7.

1. Memory. 2. Memory – Age factors. 3. Memory disorders.
4. Mnemonics. I. Wiles. Janet, 1960– . II. Australian Broadcasting
Corporation. III. Title.

153.12

Illustration Credits
Illustrations on pages 64, 119, 153, 158, 164 and 166 by Edwina Riddell.
Cartoon on page 39 by Harry Roberts.
Illustration on page 169 by Nic Geard.
Designed by Fisheye Design
All diagrams and other illustrations by Jane Cameron.

Set in Minion 11/14 pt
Colour reproduction by Colorwize, Adelaide
Printed in Hong Kong by Quality Printing

To U3A (University of the Third Age) for the wonderful way they promote ongoing challenge and the joy of lifelong learning to people worldwide.

About the authors

Judith Wiles received her Bachelor of Arts from Macquarie University as a mature-age student, majoring in Behavioural Science and Education. After she completed her studies she taught life span development at TAFE until she retired. She lives in Sydney.

Janet Wiles is a cognitive scientist and Professor at the University of Queensland. Her research centres on how the brain works. She is also co-director of the Centre for Research in Language Processing and Linguistics. She lives in Brisbane.

Acknowledgments

Our grateful thanks go to: Moira Pieterse (then President of the Sydney Northern Region of the University of the Third Age) for her invaluable assistance with our 'Survey on Memory' and to the Memory Survey respondents for sharing with us their trials and their solutions, their wish for knowledge and philosophy of self-help; Catherine Harrell, whose support and practical suggestions we value beyond measure; Sue Barker, Helen Chenery, Stella Cornelius, Jennifer Hallinan, Leanne Rylands, Judith McLeod, Ruth Schulz, Anne Smith, Dawn Wiles and Robert Wiles for variously foraging for information and insightful comments on particular chapters; and Harry Roberts and Nic Geard for their original cartoons and drawings.

Preface

Writing this book in collaboration with my daughter Janet has been a journey of great joy. I have moved from being often in a state of worry over my many small slips of memory and dread of possible worse to come, to a position of interested spectator as well as chief custodian of my memory system.

Janet and I live 1,000 kilometres apart and keep in touch by phone and email. By these means she would often share with me her excitement over her latest reading about the working of the brain. We began a series of question and answer correspondence over my memory lapses, with my worrying diminishing in importance the more I knew about it. The final result was the writing of this book.

We hope that its readers will feel pride, as we do, in being the owners of such a marvellous contrivance as the human memory system, and gain understanding of how to tend it with care and be gentle with its occasional lapses.

Judith Wiles

My mother always had a good memory. When she started worrying about her memory failing, the family used to joke that she was just having trouble getting used to living with a normal memory system. Learning about memory changed her life. What began as a simple conversation between the two of us about memory grew to be a fascination, prompting a survey about other people's concerns. Answering the concerns of the survey respondents grew from a report, to a paper, then got out of hand and grew into this book. We hope that it will be of interest to anyone who has wondered which of their 1,000 billion brain cells mislaid the car keys.

Janet Wiles

Contents

About the authors   vii

Acknowledgments   viii

Preface   ix

1 Why Do We Forget Names?   **1**
   The Memory Survey   2
   Issues from the survey   4

2 The Memory System   **10**
   Conscious and non-conscious memories   11
   The three phases of memory   17
   Why we forget   27

3 Dealing with Glitches   **31**
   Absentmindedness: glitches in encoding   32
   Forgetting over time: glitches in storage   40
   Tip-of-tongue and other glitches in recall   43
   Lighten the memory load   46

4 Improving Memory over Time   **52**
   Good organisation for the longer term   54
   Memory in social situations   60
   Unwanted memories   64
   Learning new technology   69
   Remembering numbers in everyday life   71
   Methods of the masters   74

5 Normal Ageing and Normal Forgetting   **80**
   Concepts of normality   81
   Memory for long ago   90
   Differences between older and younger people   93
   Variability in ageing patterns   100

6 Normal Memory Loss or Alzheimer's?   106
     Difficulties with diagnosing Alzheimer's   107
     Myths about memory   108
     Comparing normal changes with Alzheimer's   110
     Where to go for help   115
     Ongoing research   122
     Further information on Alzheimer's   125

7 Maintaining Health for Vintage Memories   127
     Physical and social influences   128
     Nutrition and supplements   133
     Risks and hazards   144

8 The Brain in Action   151
     Physical characteristics   152
     Cells and networks in action   156
     Different regions for different memories   160
     Current research into brain regeneration   168

9 Lifelong Memory, Lifelong Learning   173
     Incomparable memory   175
     The mind is the brain in action   177
     Memory for life   178

Further Reading   181

Endnotes   183

Index   205

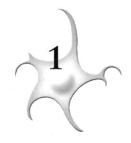

Why Do We Forget Names?

I name this ship ...
I name this land ...
I name this ~~child~~ ...
owners, great

The ceremony of name-giving is an occasion of importance and it is an honour to be asked to bestow a name. Only certain people such as the parents of a child may actually choose the name, and sometimes traditions decree who the child will be named after. So here we are, as adult people, with a name that defines us, and yet that name is an arbitrary label. Surely we would be the same people had we been called some other name. A name is not intrinsic to us, not literally part of us like a foot or a face. The paradox is that although we would still be the same person with a different name, we learn to identify ourselves by it and build our personalities around it.

Since calling others by their name is an important part of our social and business life, we would like to remember their names. Almost everyone has

1

experienced a situation where they know the name of a person but cannot bring it immediately to mind. Frequently this lapse occurs when the person has not been seen for a while but it also occurs for names of close friends and even family, or somebody met only minutes ago. Why are names so hard to remember? The arbitrary association between a person and their name provides a clue to our difficulties in remembering names and bringing them to mind at will. If words form a sequence like 'left and right' or 'warm and cosy', they come easily to mind. One word calls up the next. But a person and their name are two discrete entities and we need to deliberately create associations between the two.

Funny things can happen when other people forget *your* name. Helen recounts her story:

> At our local shopping centre a woman rushed over and said how lovely it was to see me and continued to chat for about 5 minutes. The whole time I was racking my brains trying to remember who she was – I was searching for clues in everything she said. She finally said she had to be off and said 'good bye Susan – see you soon I hope'. My name is Helen!! What a relief – she didn't know me after all!

The Memory Survey

To find out how much people were concerned about their memories, we designed a short 'Survey on Memory'.[1] Judith's local region of the University of the Third Age (U3A) kindly agreed to include our survey in a mailout to their members. Very soon our letterbox was crowded with replies, and they continued to arrive for months.

The Memory Survey began by asking 'Have you noticed any memory lapses in yourself?' and if so 'What things do you forget?' Most survey respondents (97 per cent) reported forgetting something. With mixed chagrin and good humour they described their lapses of memory, what memory issues interested them, what they could be philosophical about and what baffled or worried them.

The most frequently reported memory lapses were:[2]

- Forgetting names of people and things   179 responses (65%)

- Things to do, such as make phone calls,
  remember birthdays   77 responses (28%)

- Automatic actions, such as whether   58 responses (21%)
  doors were locked; irons and stoves
  turned off; where keys, glasses,
  umbrellas or cars had been left

Other difficulties mentioned were past events, finding the right word, phone numbers, passwords, pin numbers, information read, and words of a new language. Three per cent of survey respondents gave no memory lapses but, interestingly, only a very few claimed perfect memories. Most of the 3 per cent reported highly effective strategies for organising their lives.

Participants in the survey were also invited to recount anecdotes about memory, many of which are quoted, with permission, throughout this book using pseudonyms. The anecdotes and other information confirmed that memory failings were indeed a major issue for most of those who responded. However, for a few people they caused little worry. As one respondent wrote, 'Cease trying to recall, just let it come!' Temperament and coping skills vary, and many respondents were philosophical about memory loss.

Of all our friends, we would have said that Angus, a keen birdwatcher, was one who had no memory problems. A former managing director of a large engineering firm, he is decisive in everything he does and cryptic in his speech. One day as he sat in a large easychair, Judith commented that this is why she hadn't been birdwatching lately and handed him the Memory Survey report, then departed to the kitchen to make tea. As she returned he was running his finger down the list of items people forgot, saying: 'I do that ... I do that ... I do that ... ' That someone so intelligent and sharp would have memory lapses surprised Judith. As our study progressed, it became clear to us that minor lapses are normal for everyone. They do not indicate loss of intelligence and needn't interfere with a warm and active social life.

Memory is a much-studied topic and the scientific literature we consulted showed us that there is a plethora of information about memory. Our task in writing this book was to gather together the pertinent details scattered throughout such diverse fields as biology, neuropsychology and neuroscience. Our sweep included all the main issues raised by the Memory Survey respondents, nearly all of which related to memory for everyday living.

Issues from the survey

[I forget] names both of things and of people; facts – including facts I'd imagined I'd remember forever – I even forget scandals! Words – I often complete my sentence differently from the way I had intended because I can't recall the word I intended to use.
BEVERLEY

Names and words

Since names topped the list of memory lapses, we looked for reasons why names cause so much worry. We found two major underlying concerns:

1   The first is the embarrassment experienced in social situations, where to forget a name seems to indicate a lack of interest in the person, when in fact quite the reverse is the case. The face is familiar, the identity is known, the person is valued and we mind if they are hurt by us forgetting their name.

2   A second and underlying cause of worry is the thought, 'Is this the start of something worse, is my mind going?' Probably not. It is normal for memory to begin slipping a little from about 60 years of age (dignified in the memory literature by the term 'age-associated memory impairment'). Such slight losses do not interfere with normal living, nor do they foreshadow worse to come.

The survey showed that the majority of respondents were concerned about remembering the names of people they know well and were variously embarrassed, worried or curious about their memory lapses. For example, one respondent wrote, 'It is a nuisance to put something down and not remember where. But I can have a panicky feeling about names.' Another aspect of concern about lapses is that, at some deep level, people feel power when naming things, a view expressed eloquently by Oliver Sacks, who wrote: 'What is naming *for*? It has to do, surely, with the primal power of words, to define, to enumerate, to allow mastery and manipulation; to move from the realm of objects and images to the world of concepts and names.'[3]

Names have a huge importance in our lives, not only of people but of objects, places, books, games, tools and appliances. Names allow us to label things so we can refer to them easily. Imagine trying to chat to someone without using the name of anyone or anything. We really would be reduced to pointing or to saying what the object did or was made of. But, useful though they are, names are only arbitrary labels. Any label would do so long as there is agreement among people about what the name–symbol stands for. People who know more than one language are well aware that the same object can have many names. The processes of remembering and forgetting are explained in Chapter 2, 'The Memory System', and strategies for remembering names are detailed in Chapter 3, 'Dealing with Glitches'.

Remembering future intentions

I have gone downstairs and forgot what I came for.
CORINNE

After names, the next issue of importance to Memory Survey respondents was remembering to do something at some future time. The committing to memory of our intentions and the execution of them at the right time is an intricate task for the memory system. Very often we commit to memory the *intention* but not the means of recalling that memory when the right time comes. This kind of lapse is not surprising since intention and execution are managed from two different parts of the memory system. Unravelling the nature of the memory system is the subject of Chapter 2, 'The Memory System'. This chapter also gives explanations to exasperated Memory Survey respondents like Val, who wrote, 'There is no rhyme or reason why I can't remember some words until after the need to use them.'

What is just a memory lapse or what indicates a short-term memory failure and not just a natural forgetting?
TARA

By 'memory lapse', we usually mean a name or fact we can't think of right now but usually do remember a little while later. 'Short-term memory failure' would mean a name or fact was not sufficiently fixed in memory in the first place. 'A natural forgetting' could refer to something like the name of a town you visited on a trip 20 years ago and have not thought of since. These various types of forgetting can be understood in terms of the three phases of memory: taking in information, storing it and recalling it. Glitches can occur in any one of the phases.

Many of the survey respondents expressed wonderment that the name or whatever they were trying to remember would not surface when they wanted it, but did so hours later, or in the middle of the night, or upon waking the next morning. When someone blocks on a well-known name, the memory system has not forgotten it. Rather, the problem is one of fishing it out. In many cases the wrong word may block the right one from surfacing. Such other words are interlopers that will go away over time. Other cues, even ones we fail to notice, may then trigger the right name.[4]

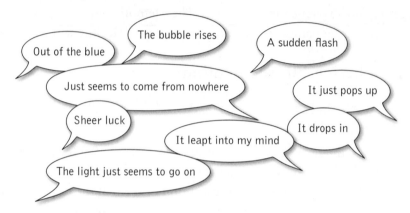

Half-joking, half-serious comments from the Memory Survey respondents in answer to the question, 'If you remember later, what prompts the remembering?'

Absentmindedness

> *They say you remember things you 'need' to remember and I'm sure this is true. But the short-term loss is getting decidedly worse – and walking from fridge to table and back gets tiring after a while.*
> **JERRY**

After forgetting names and future intentions, absentmindedness such as losing keys and glasses ranked third in the concerns of the Memory Survey respondents. A little more concentration is the answer to absentmindedness. Other types of forgetfulness need other types of strategies and are explained in Chapter 3, 'Dealing with Glitches'. All the strategies in Chapter 3 are ones that can be put to use immediately, and the best are those that take account of the way the memory system works.

Working to improve memory

> *Is there a way to exercise the brain to help it remain more agile and not hibernate?*
> **ROXANA**

Many survey respondents showed clearly that they were prepared to do some work to improve their memories. Their queries ranged from telling a good story, how to come to grips with new technology, how to forget unwanted memories to how to learn phone numbers and other numbers in everyday life, which are all issues that take time and practice to improve. We explain how to do this in Chapter 4, 'Improving Memory over Time'. All suggestions are based on explanations from the scientific literature about why they work in appropriate situations (or don't work in other situations).

Slowing down

> *I think my inner filing clerk has just slowed down a bit – she gets there in the end. I'm not sure whether something (intangible) prompts her or whether she just shuffles along and pops it out when she finds it.*
> MAVIS

Queries from the survey respondents included which lapses are normal in ageing, with such questions as:

> *Is it harder to remember names as you get older?*
> VIV

> *Is memory lapse a product of ageing – or is that a myth?*
> HEIDI

> *[I would like to know about] the development of memory loss, next to be expected and anything to retard, combat it.*
> VAUDON

These various issues are explained in Chapter 5, 'Normal Ageing and Normal Forgetting', and the outlook is very positive. Although studies show that older adults do have more difficulty than younger adults in recalling names, and in remembering the 'where' and 'when' of something they did, some parts of the memory system hold up very well. All of it can be boosted by use.

Until recent times most people thought that old age was the same as dementia. The scientific community now clearly considers that normal ageing memory lapses are distinct from the memory impairments of those who suffer from a dementia disease.

Will it get worse?

Why is it happening? How to tackle it? How not to be worried by it?
WENDY

Wendy's concern was reflected many times over in the survey responses. People were unsure if mislaying glasses or forgetting a name was caused by a dementia disease (of which Alzheimer's is the best known), or was just a normal forgetting. Chapter 6, 'Normal Memory Loss or Alzheimer's?', aims to sort out the differences. In recent times there have been enormous advances in brain imaging and understanding which parts of the brain are affected by the various neurological diseases. They are different from the areas affected by normal ageing. There are medications to delay the rate of decline and mitigate the symptoms of Alzheimer's disease for the minority of people who do contract it.

Effects of lifestyle on memory

How to prevent memory getting worse. Would a diet help?
SERENA

Several survey respondents also asked about dietary supplements or other ways to enhance memory. In Chapter 7, 'Maintaining Health for Vintage Memories' we explain how physical, mental, social activity and a healthy diet all contribute to a better memory.

Brain cells and systems

[I am interested in] the biochemistry of brain function.
What is one's mental capacity?
ETHEL

The ability to manage our memories and to plan ahead obviously needs an engine-room that generates and guards those memories. The brain is such an engine-room. And it is more. It is a multi-billion-part electrical system with a fine-tuned interactive relationship with the body it both masters and serves. There is more on this incredible system in Chapter 8, 'The Brain in Action'.

Lifelong memory

There was a lady who I referred to (to myself) as 'that lady whose name I can't remember' and every time I saw her I'd go through the same torture – until I was able to change my mindset and then it was OK.

ANTONIA

Flexibility is about making changes to our thinking and our practices as circumstances make that necessary. Attitudes, habits and knowledge all contribute to the way we manage our memories, our health and our lives. The many factors that contribute to memory are like an interlocking jigsaw. The final chapter of the book, 'Lifelong Memory, Lifelong Learning', brings together the main messages of the earlier chapters: how we explain memory to ourselves, how memory is connected to our sense of self, and the ways our actions can contribute to lifelong learning.

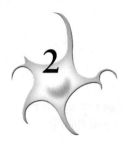

2

The Memory System

There may be no more pressing
intellectual need in our culture than
for people to become sophisticated
about the function of memory.[1]

When we have trouble remembering, why do we say 'My memory is gone'? If we have trouble walking, the doctor doesn't say 'Your walking is gone'! The doctor diagnoses a specific problem, perhaps a strained muscle. A physiotherapist may then prescribe a series of gentle exercises to tone the muscle and get it working again. The same kind of diagnosis and solution can be applied to the memory system. Much is now known about the memory system, its component parts and the intricate ways in which they interact.

How much of the complicated workings of the brain does one need to learn in order to improve memory? It turns out that a little bit of knowledge goes a long way. This chapter describes that little bit. Understanding the basics of the brain's memory system helps in managing your personal memory. You won't be exercising your arm when it's your leg that needs attention! We begin by describing the two basic memory types.

Conscious and non-conscious memories

The Memory Survey respondents noticed that they remember things in different ways. Understanding that there are different types of memory processing systems and how they work is a great tool for being more in control of one's own memory processes.[2]

The memory systems work differently depending on whether the memory is of something you *did*, some fact you *know*, or something you *know how to do*. These systems have been well researched by psychologists over a century of studies and by recent brain imaging techniques. The different memory systems can be categorised into two basic types: conscious and non-conscious.

Conscious memory

Conscious memory is the system of which we are most aware in our day-to-day lives. We know our own thoughts, remember our friends and are aware of memory lapses. Conscious memories are called 'explicit memories' and include:

- Remembering specific incidents that involved you: for example, remembering your tenth birthday, or where you put down your keys, or if you locked the back door. These are personal episodes that you experienced, and the memories of them are called 'episodic'.

- Remembering general knowledge and facts, such as people's names, the fact that sea water is salty, or that children's stories give the North Pole as the address of Santa Claus. This kind of knowledge is called 'semantic'.

Episodic memory

> *[I forget] fairly recent things: appointments; to carry out certain things such as making phone calls; making payments on time, etc; also forgetting where things have been placed.*
> **Bruce**

Some of the things people forgot worried them more than others, particularly in social situations. Personal experiences of events are retained in the episodic memory system and are encoded with information about where and when they occurred. Recalling episodic memories depends on cues or clues encoded at that time, like what you saw or heard at the time, or who you talked to. These cues would include the idea of yourself as participant, so such memories are essentially personal. Not surprisingly, small differences occur in the exact details of what people remember about the same event. We remember best the things that affect us most.

To understand how the brain recalls episodic memory, consider the following actions:

You have walked through many doors
You have greeted many people
You have given presents to many people
but ...
if you string together doing those things last Saturday at 1 pm, they become one episode called a birthday party.

The sight of the birthday person, the taste of the birthday cake, the sounds of the conversations and your pleasure in being with those people are immediately collected together in one part of your brain, called the hippocampus. However, this binding together of the parts of a memory is initially tenuous. Over the next few days, without your awareness, your brain starts to transfer it to a more permanent storage. If you also recall the events a day, a month, and a year later, they will become more firmly fixed. The complete consolidation process can take years.[3]

SEMANTIC MEMORY

Semantic memory is the intricate network of concepts and associations, facts and words that constitute our knowledge of the world. It is the focus of education, philosophy and beliefs and we carry it with us into old age.[4] The vast store of everything we know or have learned about is called 'semantic memory'. In contrast to episodic memory, we don't have to personally experience everything we know. We can learn from books, word-of-mouth, discussion groups, TV, radio, newspapers and school, or just working things out. This amounts to a really huge number of items. Semantic memory includes all the words of the language or languages we speak, as well as the way those words are put together to form sentences. An adult knows between 20,000 and 50,000 words, and their meanings are also considered semantic memory. We may not be able to produce a word as quickly as we would like, but a word once known and understood will continue to be known and understood.

Semantic memory also includes associations between items, including ones deliberately created to help remember a person's name. For example, linking the name Charlotte with a giant chocolate cake creates a pictorial and a verbal association (*ch* for Charlotte and *ch* for chocolate). Such associations are stored in semantic memory. We also know things by inference. Is the Pacific Ocean salty? Even if someone has never been there they will know that ocean water is salty so yes, the Pacific Ocean has to be salty. Semantic memory also includes abstract concepts such as justice, as well as knowledge not easily put into words, such as the sound of a particular musical instrument.[5]

General purpose knowledge about the world tends to be retained well as we age. Remembering where we have put down the keys is an example of episodic memory and is easily forgotten, but remembering what keys are for is a semantic memory task and in normal, brain-healthy ageing does not deteriorate significantly.

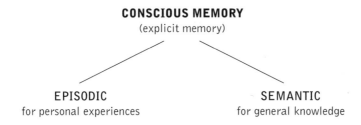

CONSCIOUS MEMORY
(explicit memory)

EPISODIC
for personal experiences

SEMANTIC
for general knowledge

Non-conscious memory

I am very interested in how the 'unconscious' mind processes conscious inquiries (e.g. names) without any authorial awareness.
NORA

A large part of the memory system is below our level of awareness. People can be influenced by recent experiences even when they are unable to recall or recognise them explicitly.[6] For example, an event earlier in our lives may have conditioned us to dislike a particular food. We do not need to remember the incident to continue disliking that food. The non-conscious memory system continually works on matters that affect us, sifting through our priorities and best interests.

Non-conscious memories are called 'implicit memories' and include:

*   Memory working below the level of consciousness, such as knowing how to do things like drive a car, play tennis or use a sewing machine.

This type of memory process is called 'procedural'. The procedure – knowing how to – demonstrates the memory. You don't need to remember when or how you learned those skills.

- 'Priming' is a type of non-conscious memory that improves your ability to remember things or objects recently encountered. Remembering happens without conscious effort.

- 'Conditioning' creates associations between previously unrelated items when they occur together or when one consistently follows the other.

PROCEDURAL MEMORY

Procedural memory is part of the implicit memory system that retains the memory of how to do things that we have already learned how to do, such as driving a car, riding a bike, or playing the piano. We do not have to remember where, when or how we originally learned and practised those procedures in order to perform them well. The *doing* demonstrates the memory.

Procedural memory is about learning skills which can become so automatic and easy to do we know them as habits.[7] For example, we have probably forgotten how and when we learned the simple skill of hand washing, but watching a small child learn is instructive. The plug is put in with ceremony, the cold tap is turned on hard, the water level rises perilously high. The soap is rubbed long and diligently between the palms while the backs of the hands remain grubby. Several tidal waves later, the soap is relinquished, the hands dipped quickly into the water, and palms wiped quickly over the towel. The small child beams with satisfaction, and the wise parent gives congratulations.

As the child is learning the skill of hand washing, he or she draws on semantic memory for facts and concepts (taps turn on one way and off the other way) and procedural memory (the many small actions involved in hand washing).

PRIMING

After recent experiences with words or objects, we have an improved ability to detect or identify them. This ability is due to a part of the non-conscious memory system called 'priming'.[8] We are not aware of the subtle changes in the brain that make recognising recent objects or words easier, more reliable or faster. It just happens.

I read a list of the names of people I expect to meet at a gathering.
TERRY

To use priming as a strategy in remembering, it is necessary to give the brain advance notice of something to be done or remembered. For example, before attending an event, read aloud a list of names and call to mind the people you've met before. Then at the event, when someone familiar is approaching you, the first name that surfaces in the memory has a much better chance of being the right one. Unfortunately, we can't use priming by concentrating and searching memory, we can only let it work. We do not feel we are remembering a past experience, but studies have shown that we most definitely can be influenced by previous experiences that we do not remember.[9] Advertisers aim to make us familiar with their products because we subconsciously prefer familiar things.

In everyday living, priming of other people's memories affects us all the time. For example, you may have put forward an idea at a meeting only to have it lapse through general disinterest. At a later stage someone from that meeting may propose exactly the same idea as your original one, quite believing that they had just thought of it themselves. Priming does not involve recollection of when or whether that idea had been encountered before.[10]

CONDITIONING

Classical conditioning is the pairing of unrelated items which occur at a similar time.[11] This was discovered by the Russian psychologist Ivan Pavlov in the early 1900s, in his famous experiments on dogs. To test conditioning in dogs, Pavlov set up an association between a bell ringing and food being provided. After the dogs were well conditioned in this way, Pavlov found that the dogs would salivate at just the sound of the bell, even when no food was given. However, the association between bell and salivating did not continue indefinitely. It faded away if the genuine reward was never given, but the association remained if the reward was sometimes given.

Mostly conditioning happens without our awareness, but there are times when we can consciously condition ourselves. Anthony Robbins, in his best-seller *Awaken the Giant Within*, tells how to lose weight by conditioning yourself to dislike high calorie foods.[12] If massive pain or disgust is associated with particular types of food there will be no temptation to eat them. Similarly, students can condition themselves to get into a study mood quickly by only using a particular desk for study. Advertisements that link unrelated items, such as beach scenes and soft drinks, are conditioning us to associate positive emotions with their products.

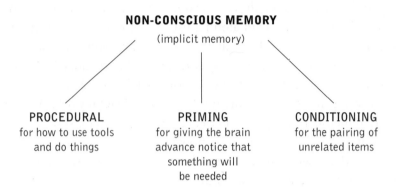

NON-CONSCIOUS MEMORY

(implicit memory)

PROCEDURAL	PRIMING	CONDITIONING
for how to use tools and do things	for giving the brain advance notice that something will be needed	for the pairing of unrelated items

Non-conscious memory and Sigmund Freud

Implicit memory is a non-conscious part of our minds, but it is different to the unconscious mind as theorised by Sigmund Freud in the early 1900s. For many decades, the only explanation of non-conscious memory was that put forward by Freud, who evolved his theory and practice of psychoanalysis based on his ideas that unconscious drives, motives and instincts govern everything people do.

Much of what Freud wrote is now outdated. The term 'unconscious' or 'non-conscious memory' is now understood and used in a different way. In the latter half of the 20th century the use of brain scans has taken our knowledge of mind and memory in great leaps forward. Many of our memory processes depend upon a relatively simple process of association, the pairing of previously unrelated items which can happen below our level of awareness (very different to Freud's emphasis on sexual urges and conflict).

The three phases of memory

Learning is the process by which we acquire new knowledge, and memory is the process by which we retain that knowledge over time.[13]

Just as there are different *types* of memory, conscious and non-conscious, there are also different *phases* that information must pass through. There are three phases of memory, analogous to putting a book on a library shelf, storing it there over time, and then finding it again later.

Many survey respondents regretted that they could not call to mind names of people just met or whereabouts of keys or eye glasses. The reality is often that the information was not put into memory in the first place. The first phase of the memory process, encoding, fixes in memory the things that we attend to.

The second phase, storage, happens below our level of awareness. If we do the encoding right, storage will generally take care of itself. However, we can strengthen how strongly a memory is stored by frequently bringing it to mind.

The third phase of the memory process, recall, is activated when we want to use the information and need to bring it back to mind. Recall is usually blamed for memory lapses, but the three phases must work together. Consider what has happened when you can't recall the name of someone you met recently: if you were not really attending in the first place and the name never got into storage at all, the problem is with encoding; but if you feel you know the name but it just won't surface right now, the problem is with recall.

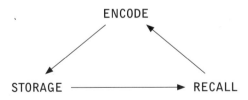

THREE PHASES OF MEMORY

A simplified diagram of the three key processes of memory: we note (encode) something, keep it in storage and later recall it.

Encoding

Encoding involves taking in information via the senses or through thinking about things. New information could be absorbed from seeing, hearing, smelling, tasting, or touching something, or using more than one of those senses. Multiple encoding is much more effective than just using one sense. Even better is adding movement, such as shaking hands. Best of all is linking the new knowledge to already known information.[14] For example, linking features of new technology to other things already well known. Specific events and general concepts both work well as associations.

YOU ENCODE WHAT YOU ATTEND TO

The memory system encodes what we are currently attending to. Since there are limits to the number of things we can focus on, attention is restricted to the things we are most interested in at any one moment.

UNDERSTANDING AIDS ENCODING

It is much easier to encode firmly and hence remember something if you understand what it's all about. How comprehensible is the following passage?

> It is probably better to do this when it's dry, otherwise things stick. A vigorous side-to-side movement is effective, as well as warming you up. However no particular technique can ensure against the whole procedure needing to be repeated at regular intervals.

These instructions would be much easier to memorise if you know that they describe sweeping a garden path! Understanding meaning is an enormous help to encoding because it enables the brain to link the new information with well-encoded ideas, via well-established pathways in the brain.

EMOTIONS ARE THE VALUE SYSTEM OF THE BRAIN

Emotions are important to encoding because of their effect on mental arousal. When we are alert, we remember better. In a study by Daniel Schacter, participants first viewed very pleasant pictures of attractive men and women and then highly unpleasant pictures such as those of mutilated bodies.[15] He found that ease of later recall is tied to high arousal rather than to which particular emotion is evoked by the picture. The stronger the emotion generated – love, fear, hate, anger, shock or greed – the better the information is remembered.

In our ordinary lives we are generally not taught to recognise which emotions we are feeling. In fact the term 'emotional' is often used in a derogatory way. However, emotions – often subconsciously – are a measure of the significance of an event or a memory to a person.

There is a large and important part in the centre of the brain called the limbic system which helps to deal with emotion, endowing memories with their emotional significance or importance. The rational and the emotional contributions of our brains are inseparable. The rational part helps us to plan and achieve our goals. The emotional part tells us what goals are worth striving for.

ASSOCIATIONS

> [To remember I] concentrate on it and try to build up scenes
> and facts around it.
> BERTHA

It is common to think of memory as a record of what has happened in the past. However, a particular experience is not just one entity but is composed of several related but separate items. The linking of the several parts of an incident can happen by intention, as Bertha describes, or as a natural process, as shown in the following example. Suppose you are a home handyman and you have just hit your thumb – hard – with a hammer. Several things happen in rapid succession: pain, the sound of swearing, feeling anger, and the sight of a bruise.

Each item is registered in the brain by a different medium:

- pain – by the nerve endings in the skin

- sounds – by the auditory areas

- anger and frustration at a job unfinished – by the limbic system

- the sight of the bruise – by the brain areas specialised for vision.

If you remember the incident some time later, the hippocampus puts together those items from the cortical areas dealing with pain, hearing, emotion and vision so swiftly and seamlessly that you remember the occasion as one incident: 'the time I hit my thumb with the hammer'.

Every item we know has several associations which link it to other items we know. Individual facts may also group into categories and either the facts or the concept can be the cue we need to access a memory. All general knowledge is linked by associations in a vast network of specific events, facts, and concepts. This linking up is very different from the way books are stored in a library. If the library acted like human memory, when you pulled a book off its shelf, strongly related books from all over the library would also be dragged after it.

Finding a memory in storage is easy if you encode it with associations to other familiar items. Suppose you have just met someone named Maurice who is wearing a blue jacket and talks about growing roses. The associations of blue jacket and roses create a network of ideas that are potentially useful cues when next you see Maurice and want to recall who he is.

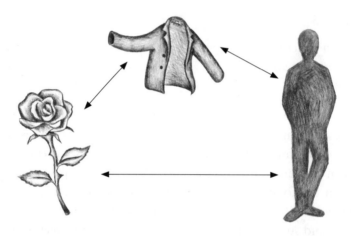

Association is a useful way of recalling names of people. For example,
a blue jacket and roses may be linked with someone you met called Maurice.

Storage

Sometimes I forget where I left an article moments after leaving it.
Arthur

Storage is essentially the preservation of memories, the all-important interval between encoding and recall. Some of these are memories we intended to keep while others – dramatic, vivid, fearful or shocking – fix themselves in our minds without us having any specific intention to keep them.

Once the information is encoded, it is kept over time without our conscious control. We cannot see it or feel it, we just know it has happened when recall has been accomplished, giving evidence that encoding was effective. Old-timers in the country used to tell stories of the days before refrigeration, and how they cooled the drinks at party time by submerging the bottles in a creek or a dam. One end of a length of string was tied around the neck of a bottle and the other end tied to a post. When retrieval time came, a pull on the string would reveal the bottle. What the bottle had been doing down there, who its bedfellows were, were unknown. The cooled, well-preserved contents were all that mattered. Retrieving a memory often has the same feel.

Storage does happen without our awareness but we can also intentionally reinforce memories by frequently bringing them to mind and mulling over them.

FROM TEMPORARY TO LONG-TERM STORAGE

All the information the senses bring in – like sounds or sights – linger only for a moment if the memory system has no reason to record them for longer. Not everything makes it into long-term storage. The brain retains only the most important aspects of the sensory input.

Suppose you are in a train and idly looking out the window. You glimpse innumerable scenes, but none that you specifically want to remember. The train travels on, and suddenly you see a house that grabs your interest, with a real estate agent's sign in front of it. You note the agent's details, and keep saying them over to yourself while you find a pencil and write them down. While you are rehearsing the name and number, the information is in the second of the storage areas, working memory (sometimes called short-term memory). Here ideas are juggled and alternatives swiftly considered. Working memory is also needed when you read, to hold on to the beginning of a sentence until you reach its end. In fact, everything you consciously want to remember must pass through working memory storage on its way to more permanent storage.

Suppose that after the train journey you call the agent, find that the house is available for holiday renting and go there with the family for a great holiday. Thinking back later about that holiday you remember the horsy smell when you went riding, the feel of the wind in your face when you walked through the hills and the hot delicious dinners. These memories are now in long-term storage.

Technically, memory researchers regard a memory as 'long-term' when it is firmly stored. This can take as little as two minutes, but the trace of the memory is still fragile at this point. Most consolidation takes place in the first few hours but can continue for up to two years. The process takes a fragile memory and turns it into a robust one, all of it happening without conscious awareness.[16]

FORGETTING MEMORIES FROM LONG AGO

Are all life's experiences permanently encoded in the brain?
NORA

Episodic memories like country holidays can be recalled with ease for about a year, and are strengthened by being frequently called to mind and spoken about.[17] The more recent the event, the easier it is to recall with accuracy and detail. As the years pass, details of a particular country holiday are forgotten as it merges with other events under a general category of 'country holidays'.

Much forgetting is normal. We would not want to keep every scrap of information our senses took in and so we rely on the memory system to filter out irrelevant information and present just the most useful information for the current moment. Forgetting could happen because the information does not pass from sensory storage through working memory to long-term storage, so it is never encoded. The memory system encodes most strongly the things given most attention.

If memory is compared to filing books in a library, then storage is when the memories are on the shelves. It's no good looking on a library shelf for a book that was never put there. But absentmindedness is not the only kind of forgetting. Do books ever fall off the memory shelves? Or just disintegrate? Can a book stay on a shelf indefinitely? A key debate for many years was whether memories stay until something else replaces them, as if they had been pushed off the back of the shelf, or whether they gradually fade and decay through disuse, like fragile material with too much sunlight on it. It's possible that both these types of losses can happen.[18] Both theories seem to agree that all our memories are not accessible to us all the time. It is not possible to know what dormant memories might be revealed if we happen upon the exact retrieval cue.

UNLIMITED STORAGE

Does one's memory become overloaded?
ETHEL

The brain has a truly remarkable storage capacity, in fact there is no known limit to the number of items it can store, but there are strong constraints on how quickly information can be added. The brain becomes tired with prolonged intense concentration and needs a short break. The sensory and working stages of memory acquisition can become overloaded if information arrives too quickly to be attended to and encoded, but items that are considered and passed on to long-term storage can continue to arrive year after year.

A firmly encoded memory is stored with its associations which act in some respects like the index system of a library, so items can be found again. But the human mind is much more versatile, intuitive and individual in the way memories are organised for storage. Associations are the links which pull the stored memories into our conscious minds.

Eyes are not camera lenses

Late in the 19th century it was believed that murder victims would store an imprint of the murderer – the last thing the victim saw – in their brains. The investigator had but to look at the brain to see the image of the perpetrator. Now we know that there could not possibly be a picture in the victim's brain. A brain is more like an electrical system than a camera. The interpretation and memory of the electrical activity is only possible to their owner. Remembering something whether it be visual, auditory or theoretical, is a reconstruction. There's no activity when the lights are out.

Recalling

*[I would like to have] some basic idea of how memory works
and the ability to recall.*

ESTHER

Recall is the return to conscious awareness of the things we have consciously
or non-consciously encoded and stored.[19] We do reap what we have sown,
not in vengeance but as the logical outcome of *how* the sowing was done.

When memory works well, we are as little aware of it as we are of our
digestive systems. However, if indigestion strikes we consciously think about
our stomachs. Similarly, when memory fails we consciously think about the
recall process.

The survey respondents reported forgetting many items, but no one
reported forgetting what telephones, keys or cars were, or how to use them.
On the face of it, how to drive would seem to be a much more difficult
concept than where the car was parked. The difference is that the part of
non-conscious memory dealing with how-to-do-things (procedural) is
very enduring. Similarly, general knowledge about keys and cars (part of
semantic memory) is also enduring. It appears that the main memory type
that lets us down is episodic – where we parked the car *this time*.

EFFECTIVE CUES

*[It's a help] remembering something else which you won't forget,
which has a link with the thing you do tend to forget.*

ADRIENNE

The key to good remembering depends on what associations were encoded
with the memory, either deliberately or by chance. Associations (or links,
cues or prompts – they all mean the same thing) are like signposts that
the brain uses to find the wanted item. When remembering a person's
name, the closer the cue is to the name, and the more associations that are
assembled, the higher are the chances of retrieving the item from memory.
The general principle is that if an item has been stored with multiple
encodings, it will have multiple signposts that can help lead back to it. Since
this does not always happen, many different sorts of cues are effective for
coaxing reluctant information from its hidden lair. One survey respondent
explained how she searches for information by 'thinking around the issue,
e.g., where did I meet that person?'

Some other effective recall techniques are:

- **The strongest recall cue is the item itself.** The best cue for a person's name is the name itself (which another person might supply for you). A name might be too weakly encoded to return by itself, or be on the tip of your tongue but temporarily blocked. If someone else says the word, you recognise it immediately as being correct. For example, 'Was his name Henry?' 'No.' 'Was it Peter?' 'Yes!' This process taps into special recognition mechanisms in the brain.

- **A segment of the original information, such as a fragment of a word.** The first syllable can be used to bring up the rest of the word. For example, a deliberate search for the name of a suburb might begin, 'Glen-something?', 'GlenGARRY?', 'No … GlenHAVEN?', 'YES!'

- **Anything associated with the person.** If you're looking at a person and trying to recall their name, any information about them is useful. 'She was looking very tanned and likes surfing – it's Robyn!'

- **The more cues the better.** One cue alone may not work. Several equally weak cues may do the trick by tapping into the right network. 'Met last week … talking about roses … Maurice!'

- **Categories.** Categories work equally well as recall cues. For example, the category 'garden' can call up 'rose'. Another item in the same category, such as a 'camellia', can also call up 'rose'.

- **Rhyme and rhythm.** Advertising jingles often use rhyme and rhythm to make their products more memorable, such as the tune for 'I like aeroplane jelly' or the sunscreen slogan 'Slip, Slop, Slap'.

The brain is very effective at combining information from completely different starting points. Consider the task of finding a mythical being that rhymes with post. 'Mythical being' is a category cue, and 'post' is a rhyme cue. In this case, the answer nearly everyone comes up with is 'ghost'.[20]

When associations do not come quickly to mind, a slow and deliberate search of memory often brings forth the memory.[21] Scrutinising one's memory involves a lengthy process of thinking around the matter to ferret out the right cues. The brain is actually assembling many different cues and may eventually find just the right association, or perhaps sheer numbers of associations will elicit the desired memory.

Searching for memory

Marcel Proust's 1913 classic account of his search to identify the taste of a little Madeleine cake reveals a determined and discerning effort:

> *Will it ultimately reach the clear surface of my consciousness, this memory, this old, dead moment which the magnetism of an identical moment has travelled so far to importune, to disturb, to raise up out of the very depths of my being? ...*

> *Ten times over I must essay the task, must lean down over the abyss ... And suddenly the memory returns. The taste was that of the little crumb of Madeleine which on Sunday mornings at Combray ... my aunt Leonie used to give me, dipping it first in her own cup of real or lime-flower tea.*[22]

MEMORIES AND EMOTIONS ARE INSEPARABLE

As we've explained earlier in this chapter, memories are encoded with their value to us (their personal relevance). When memories are later recalled, the attached feelings come too. They are an inherent part of the memory, and are re-evoked during recall. Hence, just as cues are specialised for each person, the emotions re-experienced are also specific.[23] The intensity of the re-evoked emotions can vary. When a child is describing a favourite present from their last birthday party, they are clearly reliving the joy of the moment. The memory is so vivid that it seems as if the child were back in the moment. Similarly, we might re-experience embarrassment when remembering a social event when we called someone by the wrong name. However, re-experiencing the original strong emotion isn't an inevitable process. The brain seems to have an ability to switch between remembering events directly or as if we were watching them happen to someone else. Even memories that were encoded with vibrant emotions can be recalled with weakened ones.

MEMORIES ARE RECONSTRUCTIONS

> *Memory fades with time. It is impossible to remember all the details of our lives. We have a few memories of our childhood, perhaps a special birthday party or a cross-country trip, or our*

first-grade classroom. But the details of most experiences become difficult to reconstruct as time passes. This information is not necessarily lost – it is absorbed into new experiences.[24]

Most adults remember at least some events from their childhood. Yet these memories are not like photos, a bit faded and tatty round the edges but nevertheless preserving detail accurately. This is not the case at all. A memory of a place you knew as a child is stored in the mind along with the feelings and perceptions that were present at that time. Each time you revive that memory and bring it into conscious awareness it is strengthened but also subtly changed according to your feelings and perceptions about that place now. Daniel Schacter calls it 'memory's fragile power': fragile because precise cues are required, and power because of the strength of a memory when it does return.[25] Something sad or joyous that happened 40 years ago still has power to affect us now.

Certainly our memories define who we are, however, each time our memories are accessed, details are merged into the general concept of what passed. The brain retains the essence or the gist of an episode and reconstructs details that are consistent with the main theme of what happened. As the brain accommodates new things, it alters versions of old things. New insights are added to old information, which also accounts for variations in other people's memories of the same event. As each person's life experiences are unique, so must their memories be.

Putting recall in perspective

In everyday living, recall is the most noticeable part of the memory process. It is the part that most people blame for memory lapses, even though the fault may have been through weak encoding with insufficient links to retrieve a memory from storage. But strong and appropriate links allow effective recall. Like the index system of a library, associations are the brain's signposts into memory, the words or ideas which lead to the item we want to remember.

Why we forget

[I have] odd blanks in real life. About 1961 I went by train from Port Augusta to Kalgoorlie – 3 days. My mind is a complete blank about the return journey but I presume it was by the same means.
Percy

Memory is marvellous when it functions smoothly, but as we are all too aware, it sometimes fails to deliver. Glitches occur when the memory system takes too long to deliver the information we need, refuses to deliver anything at all or delivers the wrong information.

To deal with the variety of problems in remembering, it helps to know which type of memory and which phase of the system is the culprit. The table below shows some of the possibilities for memory lapses.

Examples of lapses for different types and phases of memory

Phases of Memory	Types of memory	
	Personal experiences (episodic)	Facts and general knowledge (semantic)
Encoding	Automatic actions, such as putting down keys absentmindedly.	Not paying attention, such as not listening to someone's name when introduced.
Storage	Forgotten events that you once knew well, such as a film you saw last year.	Forgetting facts, such as exam material.
Recall	Forgetting a planned event, such as a doctor's appointment.	Knowing a fact but not being able to recall it at will, such as a name on the tip of your tongue.

Across the top of the table above are the two types of conscious memories, personal experiences (episodic) and general knowledge (semantic memory). Down the side are listed the three phases of memory: encoding, storage and recall. Thus, each cell of the table represents a particular phase of a particular type of memory. We can understand much about a memory lapse if we know which cell (or cells) of the table it belongs in. Only episodic and semantic memory are listed in the table, since they are the ones people are most aware of and therefore are most often blamed for memory lapses.

The other types of memory, the non-conscious ones, are by definition below our level of awareness, and we only know they are there by their effects, such as improvement in playing the piano after consistent practice. The phases of non-conscious memory cannot be easily separated in the way we can separate the phases for conscious memory. We can infer that glitches have occurred, but we cannot be aware of them directly.

> *I use two keys every day, one for my house, and one for the office. My hand automatically selects the last key used, which is always the wrong one!*
> Lana (a friend)

The role of priming is to help in quickly retrieving recent information. Sometimes, as is the case with Lana's keys, the most recent information is exactly what is not needed!

Another glitch in non-conscious memory occurs with motor skills. When typing fluently, we are conscious of *what* we are typing, but not the millisecond-by-millisecond synchronisation of muscles that makes it all happen. For example, one survey respondent wrote, 'When typing I am inaccurate and leave out words.' Problems with typing can occur as we get faster at the skill, and also as we age, both of which change the synchronisation patterns of the hands and fingers. One hand can become faster than the other and this requires us to consciously slow down the fingers a little, and concentrate on rhythmic or smooth typing, rather than speed.

Memory is not just one entity, but is a sophisticated system with both conscious and non-conscious parts. Not all forgetting is a glitch. An important function of memory is to extract the gist of events, and reconstruct the details. It is also necessary to forget past events in order to retain just the information we need now. For example, to remember where the car is parked today, the memory of where it was every other day is allowed to recede into the past. Memory is a balancing act between remembering what is useful and discarding everything else. The memory system mostly gets the balance right. However, when we forget something we shouldn't forget, it helps to be able to work out in which part of the memory system the forgetting occurred. We can use this knowledge to choose the most effective strategies for each lapse and understand what to do to make the strategies work.

At a glance

- The main types of memory are conscious (ones that we can be aware of) and non-conscious (ones that influence us without our awareness).

- Conscious memory includes episodic memory (the events of our lives) and semantic memory (general knowledge).

- Non-conscious memory includes procedural memory (how to do things), priming (past experience prepares us for future situations) and conditioning (the pairing of items that occur together).

- All types of memory happen in three phases: encoding, storage and recall.

- Encoding (like putting a book on a library shelf) takes in new information or re-works information already stored.

- Storage (like preserving a book and documenting where it is) holds a memory for moments (while juggling decisions) or for several minutes to a lifetime.

- Recall (like retrieving a book from the shelf) brings stored memories back to mind.

- Associations (cues) are the tags which attach during encoding, remain with the memory during storage and assist with recall.

- Glitches can happen in all types of memory at any of the three phases.

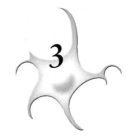

Dealing with Glitches

I would like to know some strategies or aids.
Marty

Usually we take the ability to remember for granted, until one day we realise we are forgetting things we used not to forget. This is normal. Forgetting names and mislaying keys is annoying but not medically serious. Minor memory lapses are just that (minor!), and not worrying about it frees the mind to work out strategies that will avoid the inconveniences of lapses.

In this chapter we list the most common items people forget, as reported in the Memory Survey[1], together with the strategies that respondents found helpful and those described in recent scientific literature on memory. We found much agreement between the anecdotal and the scientific sources, reinforcing our view that the best strategies are the ones that people are already using and finding effective. Building on these hints, we explain why they work and how they tie in with the memory processes of encoding well, maintaining stored items over time, and recalling easily.

One of the Memory Survey respondents said that she did not have any strategies, she just always put her keys on a hook! That *is* a strategy and a very effective one. The fact that it is very simple only adds to its value. A strategy is just a habit or plan for dealing with a particular situation. Professional memory performers demonstrate fantastic techniques but those strategies require too much training and too much effort to help with everyday practical problems. The best strategies for everyday living are the ones that people learn easily, are useful immediately and are founded on the way the brain functions. The aim is to make life comfortable and our minds sharp.

> *I have always been in the habit of writing lists and reminder notes, etc. In fact I find it is necessary for me to function efficiently.*
> *I don't often forget the practicalities of day-to-day, but I find it's not because I have a good memory but rather because of the above habits.*
> JILLIAN

Absentmindedness: glitches in encoding

The following are frequent memory lapses that are caused by not paying enough attention at encoding time:

- Forgetting new names – can't put name to face.
- Automatic actions – locking up, turning off appliances, losing things.
- Forgetting where the car is in the car park.
- Going to a room and forgetting what is wanted.

All of these glitches can be reduced by concentrating a few moments longer when you first meet a person, prepare to go out or put something down, leave the car or go to get something. It's amazing what a difference a second or two makes. During those few extra moments you need to make more than one association to create a network of links for future recall – the multiple encoding described in the last chapter. Using several senses together – eyes, voice, ears, touch, or a movement – is an excellent beginning to a new memory.

Remembering new names using mnemonics

Often there is nothing in a name that links it to its owner, and in fact the brain stores the sounds of a person's name in a different place from facts about them. This is why it is possible to recall exactly who a person is, but forget their name. Many things we know about a person link easily into a web of associations, but a link to their name is an additional task that must be created artificially.

On hearing a name for the first time some people try repeating the name to themselves which can keep it in working memory, but doesn't necessarily move it on to long-term memory, or set up appropriate recall cues for later. A technique to take the memory that one step further is to imagine the name physically attached to the person, for example, written in large writing across a head band.

Another approach is to use the sounds of the name to link in other words and images. Recall the name 'Maurice' from the last chapter. We made associations about him talking about roses and wearing a blue jacket. To ensure the name itself surfaces, imagine him pruning his very tall roses standing on bags and bags of rice and he's calling for 'More-Rice'. Images for names work best if the person is doing something exaggerated, moving, unusual or ridiculous.[2] The more outrageous the better.

If some names don't have syllables that turn easily into words, then often just the first syllable is sufficient. For example, using 'Damien' concentrate on an image of a glorious daybreak with the sun just rising and Damien furiously driving a chariot that pulls the sun into the sky.

Some names are words in their own right. Studies have shown that a name like 'baker' is more easily remembered as an occupation than as a surname.[3] As an occupation, baker has associations such as warm kitchens, loaves of rising bread and the smell of yeast. As a surname, Baker does not tell you anything about the person. A visual image could be of Mrs Baker sculpting her face in a huge loaf of fresh bread.

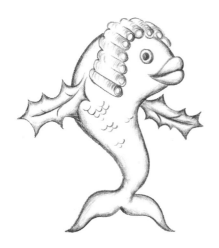

To remember a name, create a mental image that exaggerates and links the sounds of the name. For example, to remember a new acquaintance called Holly Fishwick, an image that combines all the sounds might be an exaggerated fish wearing a wig, with giant holly leaves as fins.

We had a Dr Knaggs – I told myself just think of Horse – Then I could only remember him as Dr Horse. Oh boy! The joys of getting older.

CHARLOTTE

Charlotte is definitely on the right track, but her memory let her down by substituting 'Knaggs' with the more common name, 'horse'. 'Knaggs' could be strengthened by adding a visual association. Imagine a splendid racehorse about to win a race with the camera focussed on its galloping knees. The recall pathway now becomes a mini-story of: horse–galloping–KNees–Knaggs.

These types of artificial aids to memory are called 'mnemonics'. Any catchy phrase or image that reminds you of the thing you want to remember will serve as a mnemonic.

USE MULTIPLE ENCODING

When features and items about a person have been artificially linked in your brain, recalling any one of them will bring up the others. Consider meeting someone for the first time. After you hear the name clearly, perhaps having asked for it to be repeated, think about several ways to link other features or actions to the person's name and face. Do this by hearing and looking and doing some action like shaking hands, or imagining sharing an activity, such as running a race. Even imagining shaking hands with them or writing their initials in the air just above their head creates links. Brain imaging studies have shown increased activity in the brain area concerned with movement when people simply imagined moving their hands as if to grab hold of an object.[4]

Multiple encoding provides many associations that will be useful later to retrieve a name. With attention (and some practice), the whole process can happen in the time you say 'Hello' to a new person.

REVIEW NAMES BEFORE AN EVENT

After a social event, names can be strengthened in memory by writing them down, for example in a diary, and reviewing them before the next similar function. This is also a good time to create a mnemonic for the name and an image to go with it. Writing the name helps strengthen the encoding and storage processes. Reviewing it primes the memory before future social events and builds on the way our brain naturally works. The brain does not search systematically through everything stored, as one might if one were searching through a week's supply of newspapers for a particular article. If cues form a sufficiently strong network, they fast-track the brain straight to the memory required. The brain puts most effort into quickly retrieving recent memories and memories that have been frequently called to mind. If you practise recalling names a day and a week after meeting new people you are convincing your memory that you really need this type of information.

LINKING NAME AND FACE

> *[I forget] people's names while I remember the faces.*
> HELENA

Remembering faces is quite different from remembering names. There is a component in the brain that recognises whether the face is familiar or not, another separate component that identifies who the person is and another for the sounds of their name. To an artist, the shape of a person's eyebrows matters, as does the length of the nose and the curve of the lips. Artists may well remember faces in terms of such component parts, and police identikits are based on such components. But the brain seems to have a special system dedicated to recognising faces as wholes.[5] In fact, this capability is quite remarkable. Most people can recognise up to 1,000 faces fairly easily, though this ability can be reduced by age, tiredness, stress or poor vision.

The strategy is to really look at the face for the impression it gives you. One of the Memory Survey respondents encoded faces by looking for similarities to other people he knew. Agatha Christie's famous character, the detective Miss Marple, does this to give clues on what the person is really like. That certainly would make you study the face a bit longer. We might, of course, be mistaken about a person's attributes, just by looking at the face, but our suppositions are helpful to memory by putting the person in a context. We then have the multiple associations needed for strong connection between name and face.[6]

Some people are generally better at recognising faces than others. But, surprisingly, there is little correlation between a person's estimate of how good they are and their actual ability. When you recognise a person's face, most of the process is instant, effortless and unavoidable. Remembering the faces of friends and family rarely causes a problem for the majority of people. However, recognising a face is rarely the end goal. Usually we want to attach a name as well and for this we need to go back to the strategies for names. To attach a name to a face, a firm link must have been made between the face, the sounds of the name and other identifying features about the person.

LEARNING MANY NAMES AND FACES

> *In learning the names of my large Scripture class it is easiest to learn the names alphabetically then put a face to the name.*
> VIV

When the task is to connect a lot of names to faces, such as at a wedding, in a classroom, or chairing a meeting, some prior preparation can assist. Use mnemonic tricks to learn the names from a list, then attach each name to the face when you meet the person.

Automatic actions

> *[I keep] forgetting if I have done things, e.g. close doors, turn off iron; automatic actions which I don't notice and hence don't remember.*
> WENDY

Many familiar and routine actions can be done very quickly and without having to concentrate on them at all. The 'automatic pilot' can turn off the gas and lock the back door while you are focussing on something else. Then when you are well away from home the awful doubt appears. Did you turn off the gas? Did you lock the back door? It is more than likely that you did, but these automatic actions can be very hard to recall. The same process applies to putting down keys, glasses and books. So little attention is used that the information is very weakly encoded and suffers from a lack of distinct cues because it is so similar to previous occasions.

> *It must have been me that left the book on the armchair, because it was eventually found nestling snugly down beside the cushion where I was reading it last weekend. Why don't I remember it?*
> LOUISE (A FRIEND)

Automatic actions are so easy and well known to us they become habits, a part of implicit memory.[7] Our actions continue while we think about something else, which is a great saver of memory energy. The drawbacks, however, are all too obvious. Have we done it or not? The solution to automatic actions is to focus briefly but definitely on what you are doing, giving the fleeting sensory memory a chance to move on to working memory and to long-term memory. Two seconds of attention is all that is needed to make a stronger encoding.

ROUTINE CHECKING

The process of completing a checklist is used in many jobs to ensure that routine safety procedures are not overlooked. Pilots call it a 'cockpit drill'. A drill for leaving home could be mentally running through a sequence such as 'back door – iron – stove – front door'. Because we have such a strong sense of place, it seems easier to remember movements around the house if they are always done in the same order. Then you can be sure not only that you *have* turned off the stove, but also that you remember doing so. Many people also use a very short drill before they leave home or car, such as 'pause – check for wallet and keys – shut door'.

KEEPING TRACK OF BELONGINGS

A variation of the cockpit drill works well when you are on the go, shopping and carrying parcels or travelling with luggage through airports. You are constantly monitoring your possessions, so just counting them serves as an excellent recall cue. It is easy to work out what is missing when the count falls short. Although we might not call them by this name, we use 'cockpit drills' in many situations: leaving a friend's home, collecting children from school or preparing for a picnic.

PUTTING DOWN KEYS

> *Certain places for certain articles – always.*
> CATRIONA

People who always know where their keys are don't necessarily have a good memory. They usually have a convenient, permanent 'home' for the keys and have trained themselves to put the keys there every time.

> *When I was travelling around for work, on arriving at a new place I used to choose a place for my keys, usually just inside the front door, put a stick-on hook on the wall and immediately hang my keys on it. The habit served me well (mostly).*
> TRACEY (A FRIEND)

Some people worry about keys on hooks being too obvious to burglars, but nobody knows your home as intimately as you do. An appropriate place is one where you can conveniently tuck away the keys as soon as you come in, but not be visible or reachable from outside the house.

SPECS NEED A CATEGORY OF TEMPORARY HOMES

Taking glasses off and putting them down while thinking of something else stirs so few brain cells that the action is very poorly encoded. When next the spectacles are needed, it can be very difficult to remember where they were put down. No amount of crossness with oneself stops the practice from being repeated, and no amount of good intention will cure the habit.

What does work is to select a category of acceptable places to put glasses, such as a shelf or a table which are found in most rooms. Then train yourself to hold your glasses until you can put them on a shelf or table. The strategy dramatically reduces the number of places where the specs could be if you need to search for them later. A habit that is a little harder to teach oneself, but is very effective, is to watch your hand putting the item down and note the colour and texture of the surface.

MENTAL RETRACING

> *I have a favourite cafeteria at work, and whenever I can't find my umbrella at home, the next place I look is the cafeteria umbrella stand.*
> LUCY (A FRIEND)

A friend once found her glasses on top of the pelmet in her new family room. She had been up a ladder hanging curtains. A few hours later she was frantic! She eventually found them by mentally retracing all the things she had done that day.

Mentally retracing steps involves asking oneself questions that help the memory recreate recent situations:

> When did I last have the keys? (or glasses)
> What was I doing at the time?
> What clothes was I wearing? (look in the pockets)

For any lost item, make the clues you ask yourself in the mental retracing as specific as possible to the item. For an umbrella: when did it last rain, or look like rain? For a gardening tool: in what part of the garden would you use it?

Give yourself time to ponder the answers. Additional recall cues brought to mind in this way can quite dramatically narrow the number of places the misplaced article could be. Visualisation can be done by keeping still and letting the mind retrace your steps. Alternatively, you can physically retrace your steps, pausing to let the mind dwell on each room. Visual imaging and energetic physical movement are incompatible since both use the same part of the brain devoted to spatial memory, so stopping in each room gives the brain time to think.[8]

Losing the car in the car park

There may be occasions when you jump out of the car, immediately focus on shopping, but when you return to the car park with arms full of parcels you have no idea where the car is. A good strategy is to go back and find the door where you first entered the shop. You will probably recognise that department, so you can now try the return journey of door to car.

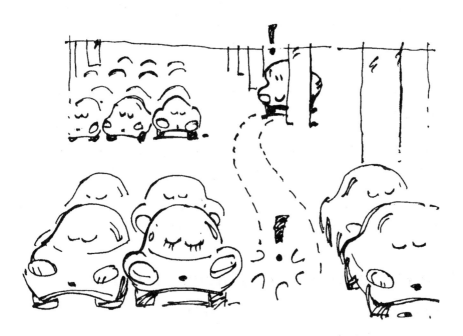

As for car parking in shopping centres – have you noticed how often the car moves when you leave it! (Ashley)

In 20 years of weekly shopping you would have parked the car a thousand times and yet you need only to remember where it is today. It is the job of the brain to forget all those other times. But for *this* time, you need to look around for good recall cues. If the floors of the parking station are differentiated by colour, stare at that colour for a few moments and say to yourself 'red floor'. If you are one of the rare people who remember numbers better than colours, repeat the number to yourself: 'Floor 4, Row G'. If it is a vast, outdoor car park, note a pair of local landmarks that you can find later. For an extra boost, as you leave the car park, turn around and look in the direction of your car and mentally visualise where it is. When you later think about returning to your car, colour or number and voice will be the multiple associations that link the car to its parking place.

Going to a room and forgetting what you wanted

> *I forgot why I have gone to the fridge or the laundry cupboard. Things I have done automatically in the past I must now concentrate on to finish the task.*
> KATYA

Sometimes we go to a certain room knowing we have to get something, but have to return to the starting point to remember what it was. The reason why we then remember so easily is that the context in which we formed the intention – the memory – is re-established. This particular form of absentmindedness can be reduced by a bit more attention to the desired article before leaving the starting point.

Interestingly, we don't usually forget which room we had to go to. Memory of place is somehow stronger than other memories.

Forgetting over time: glitches in storage

Common things people forget over time include:

- Holding on to an idea over a delay.
- Films seen recently and facts studied for exams, which are forgotten in a few months.
- Where things have been hidden from burglars.
- Names of classmates and teachers from very long ago.

The above glitches in storage can look very different, but the potential problem they have in common is the transient nature of the memories. To survive at all the memories must have been encoded, but they need to be recalled to conscious memory more often to give them strength. This rehearsal is the key to reducing the transience of such memories. Transience may be due to the memory itself decaying or losing the cues to recall, or both.

The fading of memories over time is normal, if those memories are left undisturbed in storage. The brain generally assumes that unused information is no longer wanted. If information is important, the options are to rehearse, or to write it down.

Holding on to an idea

> How can I remember to do something 10 minutes after I have thought about it when I can't attend to it immediately?
>
> UNA

The frontal lobes of the brain play a key role in the working memory system and are called in when we must actively work to maintain information across a delay.[9] If the information is only in temporary storage and we are distracted during that time, it will be lost. One friend says that he interrupts conversations to have his say because his thought will vanish if he doesn't say it immediately.

> If I am listening to somebody else talking and I have a thought that I can not express right away, I imagine holding a fishing line which is attached to my idea. As soon as I am released from the obligation of listening, I zip to the end of the cord, and, as long I have remained aware that there is a 'fish' on the end of my line, there is my original idea waiting to be attended to. This seems to work provided there has been enough time – a second or two – to entrust the idea to the fish's care.
>
> LOUISE (A FRIEND)

In those few seconds the thought is moved on from (tenuous!) working memory to more durable memory with a recall cue attached.

For dinner conversations, sages have suggested an alternative to holding on to an idea – let the thought go. If a comment or idea occurs to a person but they don't get a chance to say it and the conversation then takes a different turn, they could imagine screwing up the unexpressed idea like a little ball of newspaper and tossing it into the nearest corner of the room. If at the end of the dinner all four corners of the room have piles of little balls, then there has been rewarding conversation at that dinner party.

Films seen recently and facts studied for exams

[I forget] the author of books and films that so impressed me I was sure I'd never forget them but sadly do forget.
PAMELA

Many occasions are vivid when we experience them, and for a short time afterwards we remember a lot about them. However, over time the details gradually fade. Talking about a film, play, opera, concert or book will help to establish some main points that are noteworthy or interesting or funny. Conversations help to rehearse the material and make the initial memories stronger. Information that is learned by linking it to things already familiar is much more durable than rote learning. Later when chatting to people about a film (or book, play or whatever), start with whatever is remembered. Other people may be able to fill in some of the gaps. The brain remembers by following links, so if each person taking part in a conversation adds whatever they can remember it builds a more complete picture and each person's memory is jogged a little further.

When faced with an exam, students are renowned for studying material the night before, retaining it just long enough to answer the questions, then forgetting it again by the time the next semester begins. If the information is not linked to other things and is not revised after the exam it is no wonder it fades.

To establish strong new memories, whether of films to tell friends or in studying for exams, the three golden Rs are 'Record, Revise and Recall'. First, write it down (or type it, take a photo or make some other sort of permanent record). The act of writing something yourself forces the memory to recycle the information. Second, rehearse the material and link it to something already known. Unfamiliar material fades quickly, so revise the material within 24 hours of learning it. Third, recall the material at lengthening intervals (for example, after a week, then a month, then a year).[10]

The technique of the three Rs also works for learning new material such as descriptions of new technology or lists of words in a new language. (Chapter 4, 'Improving Memory Over Time' has more strategies for dealing with new learning.)

Remembering hiding places

Never assume I will remember.
MEREDITH

Carefully hiding small valuable items like a brooch or ring from burglars is a considered action. It is unlikely that we would toss them down as casually as a bunch of keys. We choose a really safe place, put the items there, and fully expect to remember the place. Months later, when the items are wanted, the memory can seem a complete blank. The information probably is in the memory store, but the recall cues are not specific enough.

Physical or mental retracing can sometimes stir cues from the encoding time. A variation on retracing is to imagine holding the brooch, or whatever item you can't find, as if to ponder where would be a safe place to store it. The strategy will often prompt your brain to think of the same hiding place again. The long-term solution is simple: don't assume you will remember. Note it down, perhaps in an alphabetical notebook kept in a secure place like a lockable filing cabinet.

Names from long ago

Information from long ago will generally fade after a period of time if it is not brought to mind occasionally. Old memories of classmates and teachers may reawaken with appropriate cues. The strongest cues are seeing old friends again in person or in photos and hearing their names, and these will almost always bring to mind other friends and times spent together. A group of people sparking off each other can revive memories not thought of for years, as well as being great fun.

For accurate detail and really important information, the only sure way of remembering is having written records, with names and dates recorded.

Tip-of-tongue and other glitches in recall

One of the most embarrassing situations can happen when you know a person really well but just at the moment of needing the name it won't come to mind. Given time you will think of it, maybe in two minutes, maybe in two hours, but that of course is too late. The name feels familiar as soon as somebody else says it. We almost never truly forget the names of people we know well. Far more often the name is just temporarily blocked.

[It worries me] not remembering friends' names when
I meet them unexpectedly.
Viv

Tip-of-tongue (T.O.T.) is the frustrating experience of knowing a name or word but not being able to produce it at the moment it is needed. You have the feeling that the name is hovering just out of reach. People of all ages experience it. In fact, it is such a universal human failing that almost every language has a phrase for it.

The T.O.T. phenomena happens on average once to twice per week for college students and two to four times per week for older people.[11] It usually happens when the word or name is not frequently used, but it can happen when you are about to introduce someone you know quite well. The matter is further confounded by incorrect but similar words popping into mind. These closely related but wrong words have been called 'ugly sisters' from the folk tale of Cinderella and her two ugly stepsisters who jostled her aside to try to gain the attention of the prince. We tend to dwell on these almost-right words because of the feeling of familiarity, but in fact focussing attention on them only blocks the right word from surfacing. If attention is diverted to something else, anything else, like the second best word or other things known about the person, the Cinderella word may pop up or else surface later.

Another type of blocking that feels very different from T.O.T. is a recall glitch that results in a complete blank. Nothing comes to mind and there is not even a glimmer of a lead.

Similar strategies work for both T.O.T. and other forms of blocking. The most effective method to prevent blocking is to prime the memory before social events. Such priming wakes up the related web of associations and speeds name recall, but it won't prevent blocking from ever occurring. At the critical moment, we can either search around the blockage or let it subside.

Go through the alphabet

[I use the trick of searching] for people's names by getting the first letter and fishing out names with that letter. It often works for people. Not objects or concepts. For those I must stop from getting annoyed with myself and put it out of my mind – then it frequently pops up totally unexpectedly.
Anita

When trying to remember a familiar name and being faced with a blank, the most popular strategy cited in the survey was to try the letters of the alphabet for fit. The conscious brain can frequently recognise when we come to the beginning sound that seems right.

This method works because it taps into the way the brain responds to the initial letters or sounds as recall cues for names and provides a systematic way to search around a blockage.

Work around a blockage

> *[It worries me] seeing someone I know and haven't seen for a while and knowing I have only a few seconds in which to remember the name.*
> TARA

When you are talking on the phone or about to introduce a person and there's a blank where the name should be, you may feel pressure to respond quickly. There isn't much time but there is some. The electrical/chemical messages that travel along the nerves of the brain do so at 100 metres per second, so one or two seconds can be enough to search for some context to the person, which could bring links to the name.

> *There is no need to think quickly. Pause and think slowly instead. Pause and reflection go together.*
> EDWARD DE BONO[12]

Pausing is a good stalling technique to give your brain time to respond. Focus on something positive and achievable. If you can't think of a person's name, what do you know about them? Think about their house, their family, the way they dress, something they said, where you last met them. Work systematically through the categories of your life: family/friends; street/local/community; work, previous/present; health/hobbies/home. Daniel Schacter calls this process 'scrutinising memory', demanding that it works a bit harder and deeper.[13]

Ask other people

In a social or business group there are sometimes opportunities for getting help from other people. There is comfort in quickly asking the person next to you 'Who is that?' Then you either have the answer or at least have an ally in your memory lapse. Remember that two out of three respondents in our Memory Survey reported memory lapses for names, so you are in good company.

Lighten the memory load

It was a Sunday afternoon, about 5.00 pm. The doorbell rang. I descended the ladder and in paint-spattered clothes and paint brush in hand opened the front door. Our friends stood there in their Sunday best, carrying a bottle of champagne. They had come to dinner in reply to an invitation we had made three weeks before. My wife was at work, nursing. I am not sure who was surprised more, me or them. However, they were understanding and we ended up having a very pleasant evening after I rustled up some food and picked my wife up from work. This was about 20 years ago, and although I have forgotten some appointments since, none have seemed so embarrassing. We never used a diary in those days.
NIGEL

The Memory Survey contained many instances of forgetting to do something at a future time, such as:

- Missing social engagements and forgetting appointments.

- Forgetting birthdays and special occasions.

- Forgetting to deliver messages or to post letters.

- Leaving coats and umbrellas in restaurants.

These are all cases of forgetting something we intended to do (which is known as prospective memory). The particular difficulty in remembering future events is that the memory might be well encoded, but the recall cue needs to surface at just the right time to alert us to take a particular action.

The two key strategies for improving memory for future commitments are to:

1 Relieve the memory of as much information as possible by using written aids such as lists and diaries (recording).

2 Set up reminders such as alarms or putting letters to post by the front door (reminding).

Written aids

Writing something down is half the battle in remembering it for the future. The other half is remembering to look at what you have written. Where you have made the record and how you keep it are important to good organisation of prospective memory. The choice of record depends on how long the written records need to be kept – temporarily, semi-permanently or permanently.

TEMPORARY WRITTEN AIDS: LIST MAKING

> *I now make lists for shopping, banking, etc, but often 'forget' them at home. Nevertheless, by making the lists, it seems to be an aid to remembering the items.*
> **HEIDI**

List-making is a good thing. Contrary to the belief that list-making will make memory lazy, making a list helps to focus attention on the items and encode them better. The physical act of writing does more than create a visible record: it makes strong associations. Many items on the list could probably be remembered without looking if the shopper is the writer of the list. However, the list only lessens memory load if we check it at the right time.

Other suggestions by the survey respondents included Post-it notes, pad and pencil by the phone to write things down immediately, a white board for urgent and important things and a writing pad for so-so ones. An important part of lightening the memory load is to throw out the notes when the job is done and transfer information that needs to be saved, such as phone numbers, to a more permanent store.

SEMI-PERMANENT REMINDERS: DIARY AND NOTEBOOKS

> *As for dates and special events etc I must have my diary –*
> *I could not function properly without it.*
> **ANTONIA**

Diaries are an ideal medium for noting future events. For diaries to be effective, they generally need to be looked at every day and need a regular 'home' – somewhere handy, such as near the telephone or on the breakfast table.

Other semi-permanent types of records are health ones. Many doctors carefully describe to a patient details of the present condition, treatment and next visit. Such detailed information given in a short space of time can be hard to remember later. Many people use a small notebook in which they record all medications currently being taken and any questions they want to ask. The notebook can be taken to all medical appointments, and used for writing down the answers during the consultation.

Permanent Records: Addresses and phone numbers

An address and phone book takes some effort to write and keep up to date, but then it becomes a genuine memory-sparing device. A small booklet can travel around with you if necessary. Since a much-used item like this can easily be mislaid so it needs a home, such as near the phone, or a category of resting places as for spectacles. Some diaries have a removable section for addresses and birthdays that can be transferred from year to year.

Setting up reminders

> ... he inserted his hand mechanically into the back pocket of his trousers to obtain his latch key. Was it there? It was in the corresponding pocket of the trousers which he had worn on the day but one preceding. Why was he doubly irritated? Because he had forgotten and because he remembered that he had reminded himself twice not to forget.
>
> JAMES JOYCE[14]

Future memory tasks are of two forms: time-based (e.g. ring Sue at 4 pm) and event-based (e.g. when you see Tom, give him the article). Both need a deliberate setting of associations tied to something concrete that you will notice at that time. Intention alone is not enough!

Our perceptions of how quickly or slowly time passes are often geared to the degree of interest in present activities rather than what the clock shows. If we need to make a phone call at a certain time later in the day, we need to be aware of the passing of exactly that much time. Something in our head has to go 'ping' when the allotted time has passed (and there were many survey reports rueing the lack of an inside-head ping-clock).

> I use an electronic voice organiser (rings an alarm at predetermined times, minutes, days or weeks ahead).
>
> MILO

An event can be changed from time-based to event-based by using tangible reminders such as watch and clock alarms, electronic voice organisers, digital assistants (such as Palm pilots) and telephone wake-up calls.

Another type of concrete reminder, useful if medications need to be taken at certain times every day, is to put the medication with something you are not likely to forget, such as mealtime necessities or a toothbrush. Sometimes it is helpful to have a week's supply doled out into special containers with seven small compartments (which can be bought at pharmacies).

Another event-based cue is to put library books by the door so the sight of them when leaving is the prompt to take them with you. This tactic should be helpful but is not infallible. We heard of one shopper who carefully stepped over the books as she left. (She now reports that she has another place dedicated to the assemblage of items to be taken when going out, and this strategy works.) Another visual prompt is to put something unusual in the middle of the kitchen floor. You see it and think, 'What's that doing there? Ah yes!'

With external reminders, people of all ages can be very effective at remembering to do things at a specific time (incidentally, older people tend to be more reliable as they are often better organised than younger ones).[15]

VISUALISING FUTURE ACTIONS

Earlier in this chapter we described visualising a person with their name written on a head band. Such imagining can also be used for remembering future events. For example, to remember to take letters to post when leaving home, imagine yourself going towards the front door, and exaggerate in your imagination the act of picking them up (such as your hand sweeping up a giant letter). The strong association with the movement of your hand is a powerful reminder when you later move towards the door. The more vivid the visualisation, the stronger the mental reminder will be.

Juggling multiple tasks

I find the lack of ability to handle/consider multiple tasks and decisions at one time a real worry. The 'I can cope with only one thing at a time' is becoming very frustrating. When I was younger, handling multi-tasks was so routine.

KATYA

Many Memory Survey comments related to losing the ability to handle multiple tasks or maintaining good habits when rushed. A mental or written priority list is one way to deal with multiple tasks. Only one item can be at the top at one time, but all must have their turn of your undivided attention. The solution is to do one thing at a time and mourn the passing of the ability to do three things at once.

The ability to juggle multiple tasks is reduced if a person is extremely tired, for example caring for a sick person or not sleeping well, or is a student with a deadline for a big assignment. The ability is also known to diminish with age.

> *I have realised I have worst memory losses when I am rushed, and have numerous tasks to perform in a hurry. This may result in my placing items in completely inappropriate places.*
> LESLEY

Good habits such as always keeping keys in the same place can come under stress when unexpected things happen, or when a person is extra busy and rushed. If a regular routine is disturbed, good intentions are severely tested. One strategy is to build more time and awareness into daily activities. Stress is known to interfere with memory, so keeping calm is important. Even better is humour. To find something to laugh about is the perfect antidote for stress.

> *Make each day a new day. Take moments to ensure the things to do in the day are realistic and achievable. Allow time for self-talk. Stop pressing alarm bells by saying darn, I should have done so-and-so.*
> LIAM

At a glance

- The role of memory is to encode and store what we need and what we ask it to recall. It also has the job of forgetting everything else.

- Strategies can assist each of these stages. Which strategy is effective depends on which phase of memory is involved.

- Strategies for absentmindedness centre on creating habits that give an extra bit of attention at encoding time.

- Strategies for forgetting over a period of time centre on rehearsal (calling the information to mind more often) and searching for additional associations from encoding time.

- Strategies for glitches in recall involve giving the brain extra time and providing ways to systematically search for multiple associations.

- Strategies for remembering future events involve lightening the memory load by using lists and other written records and setting tangible reminders.

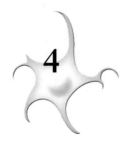

4

Improving Memory over Time

[I] would very much like to know why some people have a good memory and how to get one.
Tammy

Many Memory Survey respondents said they would like to have improved memories. There was little mention of exams and none of super-feats, just better memories for everyday living. In the previous chapter we discussed strategies for immediate use but there are some types of learning and memorising that need long-term practice. Examples include: being organised, improved memory in social situations, handling unwanted memories, learning new technology and remembering numbers.

In these cases the strategy involves managing time and effort to your best advantage. The memory system will not jump to your intentions when you say 'I really want to remember this!' any more than your muscles act when you tell them that they should grow strong and fit. To improve your ability to remember names, practise names; for numbers, practise numbers. Challenge your memory with something you really enjoy and want to learn.

'Is memory something we have or something we do?'[1] If we think about it as something we do, then plans and strategies and good organisation are essential parts of good memory.

Four steps to improving memory over time

Learning new material, new habits or new skills involves four major steps based upon how the mind naturally functions.[2] The strategies in this chapter are ones that take some effort and are best learned over time. Each involve these four steps:

1 Motivation – focus on reasons for learning the new material:

> Decide on your major memory concerns.

> Find out which strategies are appropriate.

> Choose one and begin.

2 Concentration – give the matter your undivided attention:

> Focus resources and attention on the task.

> When attention wavers bring the mind back to the point.

> Take a short mental rest when the brain becomes tired.

3 Organisation – structure material so it is meaningful for you:

> Divide the task into manageable portions.

> Link the material to things already known.

> Find the methods that suit the task and work for you.

4 Practise – add and revise new material in manageable portions:

> Practise remembering the item or the skill many times.

> Use the new item or skill in its normal context.

> Revise again a day, a week, a month later.

Good organisation for the longer term

In one time-management course we attended, the coordinator began by saying that half the population prefer one system for managing time and the other half prefer another. However, 97 per cent of the people who write time-management books are from the first group! They are the ones whose natural inclination (or compulsion) is to sit down at the beginning of a day, make a plan and then follow it through. The coordinator was one of the rare 3 per cent of gurus who didn't do that. Those in the second group also make plans, but having made a plan, they have a mental map of the territory they want to cross. They then throw out the plan and follow the map. To the first group they look disorganised and as though they are constantly not completing projects because they have mapped far more than they will ever achieve. But to them the first group explore very little of the big exciting world, and find it hard to adjust to rapidly changing situations. By the end of the course it was clear that both types are equally valid, but many of us at the seminar decided that we would prefer our accountant to have the straightforward skills of the traditionally organised group, and the pilot of any plane we were in to have the quick reflexes and rapid adjustment skills of the second group.

In reality, what works for one person might drive another to distraction. A wide range of organisational systems is available for different situations and different people.

Principles of good organisation

We all have collections of items that are (to a greater or lesser extent) organised:

- kitchen – plates, utensils, cutlery, food and recipe books

- garage or shed – tools, leisure and sports gear

- living room – CDs, tapes, videos, games and books

- office – documents, letters, photos and maps

- bedroom – clothes and shoes.

The list could go on and on. Perhaps we have never thought about these collections as organised (or disorganised) systems. But they are, and how we set them up can relieve the stresses and strains of memory. One survey respondent described how he cured his tendency to lose tools by putting up a pegboard and training himself to always put the tools back there. 'Knowing' the category of an item means knowing where to look for it, which is much easier than remembering each item separately.

There are two simple principles of good organisation, developed by studying how busy executives work at their desks, but equally useful for making a morning cup of tea or organising a workbench:

1   Easy to file and easy to find. Putting things away should be quick and easy, and the most frequently used items should be the easiest to file and to find again.

2   Fingertip management. When standing or sitting at a kitchen bench, workbench or desk, all the major items should be within easy reach.

One woman had a new kitchen built, and after six weeks was very unhappy with it. It was more difficult to make even a simple cup of tea than in her old shabby one. Eventually working out what the problem was, she reorganised the electric jug, cups, tea, coffee and sugar to all be within easy reach (a fingertip management system!) and finally got around to enjoying the revamped kitchen.

Varieties of organising systems

I have also tried to be more organised and methodical – (this goes very much against my 'normal' grain) by attempting to store and file things. This does not always work as I forget where I have 'stored' things.

ADA

Designing good systems is a skill. The secret of fingertip management is how often items are used, and how important it is that they be accessible quickly. There is a balance between how easy it is to put something away, and how easy it will be to find it again later, which is constrained by the number of items in the collection and the space available.

•   Heaps are unordered collections of small numbers of like items. Adding things to a pile is quick and easy, and the search time is not too long. For example, toys in a toy box, small CD collections, tools in a tool box. A heap is not necessarily untidy. For example, CDs might be neatly stacked but not be in alphabetical order.

- Larger collections usually need some form of organisation. For example, large CD collections often have similar types of music stored together, or are alphabetically ordered. For documents, organisational equipment includes filing draws, folders and shoe boxes.

Effective filing categories need to be easy to remember and make sense for the person (or people) using them. Alphabetical order is obvious, with each category filed under its appropriate letter: I for insurance, M for medical, and so on. This system is appropriate for documents that are only needed every few months or years. Other hanging files of a cabinet might be organised in time order: for example, with the most recently used ones at the front. This system makes sense if the most recently accessed files are also the ones most likely to be needed in the near future. Filing systems that gradually grow over time are often of this sort. The more people who use the files, the more regular the system needs to be.

Successful organisation takes into account the fact that some items from a collection may be in use, and others are being added. Hand tools will be with the handyman around the house, or on the workbench. Papers that have yet to be looked at will be on the desk, and those dealt with but not yet filed will be in a to-be-filed spot, such as on top of the filing cabinet. For collections that we use a lot, such staging places seem to crop up inevitably, so it makes sense to plan for it.

Good organisation is a great strategy to assist memory, but needs to take into account personal styles. Both heaps and neatly arranged stacks have their place. Some more ideas for better organisation include:

- A small exercise or 'house book' is useful for recording repairs to be done and tradesman's visits.

- People who travel often have a generic list of clothes to check for packing. It can be modified over time. If luggage is lost, airlines require a list of everything in the suitcase and a packing list is a useful memory aid.

- A digital camera can be used to make a quick record of everything in a house for insurance purposes.

- CDs can be arranged on top of a photocopier and their spines copied to keep a record of the collection.

- A driver's licence number can be engraved on the back of valuables. (The local Neighbourhood Watch or police station often have engraving tools to borrow.)

- For chronically disorganised clients, some accountants provide a shoe box for saving receipts and all other paperwork related to their financial affairs. They then take it to the accountant to be organised once a year.

- One colleague used to set aside a Saturday every six months to organise her files at work, taking stereo and beer to keep her company.

Organising conflicting ideas

> *Don't own too much stuff!*
> D & J (ADVICE FROM FRIENDS WHO RECENTLY MOVED)

Anyone who has moved house knows that it taxes one's organisational powers to the limit. Lists play a major role in organising ideas and reminding us of what and when things need to be addressed. They provide a way to boost our prospective memory for all stages of packing and moving.

An exercise book is useful to plan for the move and collect together relevant phone numbers and other information. An arch-lever folder with plastic sheet inserts can be used to collect relevant documents. Removal and rental companies often have checklists and tips about the stages of moving, change of address checklist, and tips on packing and dealing with removal companies.

There are many tips and tricks to making the move itself less stressful, such as labelling all boxes and packing a survival kit with electric kettle, tea, coffee, biscuits, aspirin and diary. One couple we know stays in a motel the first night.

How can memory cope with the entire relocation of one's every possession? The stress of moving for many people is not just in juggling a thousand tiny details of the move, but in organising a new life in a new place and re-establishing social networks, shopping routines and professional advisers. It is particularly stressful if the move is unwelcome.

Moving checklist

One month before

- Plan the stages.

- Notify the gas and electricity companies for both the new and old places.

- ...

Two weeks before

- Start packing non-essential items, clearly label all boxes.

- Arrange for mail to be forwarded; notify friends of new address.

- ...

A few days before

- Keep packing.

- Organise cleaning.

- ...

On moving day

- Double check cupboards, shelves, garage and loft.

- Carry important documents and valuables with you.

- ...

After arriving at new home

- Renew driver's licence and vehicle registration.

- Open a bottle of champagne.

- ...

Often there are conflicting goals and constraints, such as which furniture to keep when it is all special. To sort out confusing and complicated ideas, what is required is an aid for planning that first helps to get the ideas and their relationships in perspective. One simple technique is to write all the ideas and constraints spread out over a large sheet of paper and draw links between the main items. The technique creates a 'map' of the ideas that need to be sorted out, and such diagrams are called 'concept maps' or 'mind maps'.

Creating a concept map

Creating a concept map is the opposite process to creating an orderly list: you don't have to rank or classify first. If pros and cons keep jostling for attention in your mind and you don't know where to start, that's fine by a concept map. Start anywhere.

1   Begin by writing the main idea (such as 'Moving House') in the middle of a blank sheet of paper. Then all around it write down other ideas, drawing connecting lines back to the main idea. Keep adding ideas and links in any order, anywhere on the page. In this first stage you are just piling the ideas down on paper in any order. Keep writing until the well has run dry.

2   The second stage involves identifying key issues and circling related items using different coloured pens, which helps the brain 'see' which items go together. For example, 'furniture', 'size of rooms'. Add more items as they come to mind, and link them to the main thing they relate to. At this stage it is often helpful to write a second, clearer version of the map.

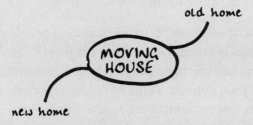

A concept map is very easy to begin: start by writing the main task to be done, such as 'Moving house', in the centre of the page; then add major considerations, e.g. the old and new homes. Build on the map by adding other things to be done or decided, drawing connecting lines between each new item and related ones.

Concept maps are actually very quick and easy to do once you have had a few practices. Since everyone's ideas and connections to other ideas are individual to themselves, a concept map is useful first and foremost to its creator. This means maps don't have to be neat and tidy but they do need to follow the basic format of putting ideas and links down first, followed by grouping associated items to impose some order.

As with the other strategies of writing down information, concept maps free the mind from the necessity of simultaneously remembering everything that needs to be done and deciding what is the best thing to be done. They provide a different type of memory assistance than do lists because they spread in all directions over a page and show the many links between interconnecting ideas. A concept map is a way of providing your brain with extra working memory capacity. Tony Buzan in *Use Your Head* gives more details on concept maps.[3]

Memory in social situations

How can one practise improving memory?
OSCAR

Improving memory in social situations is a balancing act between how much you mind forgetting things and how much trouble you are prepared to go to.

Gradual improvement in remembering names

Many of the Memory Survey respondents wanted to improve memory for names. The following three habits help to train memory for names, more as a way of life than as a course of study:

1   Prepare for social events by reviewing names of people you will meet (and mnemonics for their names if you use them). Think of the good times when you last saw these people, the things that matter to them, their families, jobs, hobbies. Think of the conversations you might have, and what you can contribute. Call to mind what you have done since last meeting them. Look up the name of a book you are reading or a film you saw. As we have explained, all these activities prepare your memory to use such information in the near future.

2   Enjoy the event. Relax, have a good time. Probe your memory calmly for the names of each person you know. If names don't come to mind

immediately, be tolerant with yourself about lapses. Find ways to use the names that you do remember. If you have a moment to spare, look at a person and silently rehearse their name. If it doesn't come to mind, don't stress yourself, but rather think of the many things you know about that person. Then mentally move on to another person and repeat the exercise. Reward yourself for your successes with a mental pat on the back. Later, return your attention to names you have forgotten. Remember that the memory system is trained by the number of times it is requested for the information, rather than intense effort in a single act of remembering.

3   Afterwards, re-live the event – within the next 24 hours have a conversation with someone, make a phone call, write a letter or write in your diary about the event and any names you can remember. Let your mind wander over the event – the people, the conversations, the food – whatever aspects interest you most. Make notes in your diary. Not only will such reliving help to fix the memories of the event, it will also help train your memory to encode similar information at the next event.

Telling stories, jokes and anecdotes

> *There is nothing worse than getting 3/4 of the way through a joke you are telling and finding you can't remember the correct sequence of the finish.*
> CON

Humour has benefits for all sorts of tensions that impede memory. It is part of human nature to enjoy telling and hearing a good story (including all kinds of anecdotes, jokes and incidents that we remember and tell to others). Many Memory Survey respondents regretted that they could not depend upon their memories to tell an anecdote without losing their train of thought. Storytelling requires more effort with age because it is more difficult to maintain focus in the face of distractions. Many people have never practised the art of storytelling. Learning to tell stories takes a little time and practice to become proficient but anyone can learn.

> *I can never remember jokes unless I jot it down first … get into the part, like an actor. I find that if I am with other people telling stories, you spark off each other.*
> RONNIE

Most people who have a joke to tell write them down in a notebook as they find new ones (even if they don't admit it!). They also practise a new joke until its delivery is smooth. Telling a story repeatedly ensures that it is encoded strongly and can be brought to mind quickly when needed. Before telling a joke, many people mentally rehearse, running through the main points to make sure each one follows easily. This process primes the memory to produce each part of the story on cue. And they enjoy the telling. There is a special magic in captivating an audience with a good story.

Just Joking

Sherlock Holmes and Dr Watson went on a camping trip.

After a good meal and plenty of wine they lay down and went to sleep.

Some hours later, Holmes awoke and nudged his faithful companion:

Watson, look at at the sky and tell me what you see

After some grumbling, Watson replied, *I see millions of stars.*

But what does that tell you Watson? asked Holmes

Watson pondered for a moment: *Well it tells me many things —*

>   *Astronomically, it tells me that there are millions of galaxies.*

>   *Astrologically, I observe that Aries is in ascension.*

>   *Horologically, I deduce the time to be approximately three-fifteen.*

>   *Theologically, I believe that God is all powerful and that we are small and insignificant.*

>   *Meteorologically, I suspect that tomorrow will be a fine day.*

He then turned to Holmes and asked, *Why did you wake me? What does it tell you?*

My dear Watson, said Holmes, *you've missed the main point! Some bastard has stolen our tent!*

Courtesy of Ronnie

ASIDES AND INTERRUPTIONS

I have learned from repeated problems not to start telling long stories of some experiences of mine as I find that, if I deviate to enlarge on some remark, when I have finished with the aside my mind has gone a complete blank and I have no recall of what I was talking about in the first place. I usually cover my embarrassment by laughing and saying 'It's all gone. I must be an early senile dementia!'

FRIEDA

When giving speeches and talks (or in fact any time) people of all ages can experience 'senior's moments', times when the brain seems to go blank and one loses the plot completely. Brain imaging has shown that such events can coincide with a physical phenomenon called a 'slow wave' moving over the frontal cortex. It is rarely possible to recover the lost state. Similarly, if someone is telling a story and has meandered into a dead end, the chances are that the departure point was not in working memory long enough to be encoded. The solution most used is external props such as finding one's place in the notes if it was a speech, or asking listeners where one was up to.

TELLING THE SAME STORY AGAIN

[I worry] that I have already told a friend what I find myself about to repeat. I ask him to stop me if I have.

CLAUDE

It is very hard getting a laugh from the punchline if your listeners heard it from you last month. A solution is to begin, 'Have I told you the story about ...?' and be ready to bridge the ensuing silence if the answer is yes.

Older people are increasingly prone to forget who they have already told a joke to (which calls on episodic memory). Accuracy for such sources can be improved by taking a little more time to search memory for distinctive details of the occurrence.[4]

Unwanted memories

I find some memory recall more unnerving than forgetfulness.
NORA

How do we forget when we want to forget? Many people have some recurring memories that cause them to feel again the embarrassment, nervousness or difficulties of a long-past situation. These are the events in our lives that we could have done without, and the recurring memories of them damage our self-esteem and our confidence. This section describes self-help techniques to help dim these nuisance types of memories and also briefly reviews the more traumatic forms of recurring memories.

The reason unpleasant memories return is powerful encoding with a strong emotion attached, and a cue that triggers the memory. Add to the recipe the habit of often thinking about the disagreeable occurrence, and that memory will be well entrenched.

One of the surprising things about the brain is the inevitability of feelings becoming attached to any memory that involves a personal experience, that is, an episodic memory. Western culture values reasoning abilities but downplays emotional evaluations. However, the brain stores experiences not just as records of events, but also with emotional significance, which is necessary for judging the importance of events. Both reason and emotion are essential to quality of life and are governed from different parts of the brain.[5]

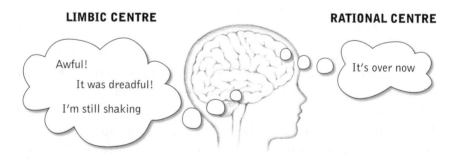

Different parts of the brain control reason and emotion. Unwanted recurring emotional memories loom larger than calm comments from the rational brain areas.

When dealing with unwanted memories there are both deep and shallow approaches that might help.[6] Addressing the underlying reasons why the memories surface is the preferred option, but in some cases treating the symptoms directly can bring relief. Below are examples of how you can do this. If the unwanted memories continue to be distressing, professional counselling is recommended.

Talk back to the internal critic

Recurring memories sometimes reflect underlying issues that when addressed, will also resolve the unwanted memory.[7] The technique of 'cognitive behaviour therapy' can be helpful to tune up a person's outlook. Consider the following examples:

- A perfectionist got a B in an exam and considered herself a failure.

- A shy young man was turned down when he asked a girl for a date and concluded that he would be lonely all his life.

- A woman forgot the punchline of a joke she was telling and thought that she was a social flop.

Some unwanted memories surface because a person is thinking in an illogical, negative manner. This often happens when someone is depressed or anxious. Psychologist David Burns collected a list of ways that thoughts can be illogical, including all-or-nothing thinking (if your performance is not perfect then you conclude that you are a total failure); overgeneralisation (a single negative event is seen as the way things will always be); and rejecting positive experiences by saying that they don't count. There are many such thought patterns which he calls 'cognitive distortions'.[8]

With a little effort it is possible to straighten out the twisted thought patterns. The approach involves recognising the illogical content of one's own thoughts. For example, if after a social event, an unwanted memory surfaces with the thought, 'I *always* make a fool of myself', this is an example of overgeneralisation.

To change perspective on a memory it is necessary to get a clearer view of what happened, to bring it out in the open to show up the wrong impression given by over-general statements. For example, writing a description of the event, or discussing it with a friend. Be specific about the memory. To write, for example, 'I was not careful enough with (someone's) name' helps to distinguish the event from sweeping statements like 'I am a social failure'.

Cognitive therapy emphasises that our feelings are created by our thoughts, not by the event itself. When over-general statements surface, talk back to the internal critic and correct the cognitive distortion. For a mental tune-up on straight thinking, see David Burns' easy-to-read description in *Feeling Good: The New Mood Therapy*.[9]

Disconnect the emotions from the memory

Consider this scenario: At a dinner party the hostess was carrying a large china dish from the kitchen to the table. She tripped over a rug and with an enormous crash, the food went everywhere. Over the next few weeks that scene replayed itself over and over in her mind. Years later it still intruded whenever she saw a similar rug or food.

When we remember events from the past we can do it in two different ways. It is possible to remember events as if we were re-living them (in the first person or subjectively) or as if we were watching them (in the third person or objectively). When we remember in the first person, the same emotions as we felt at the time are rekindled. Happy events bring back feelings of joy, embarrassing ones make us hot under the collar all over again, fearful ones make our heart beat faster. By contrast, when we remember events in the third person, we see events as an observer and don't re-live the emotions so intensively.

Some people tend to remember happy events in the first person, those wonderful times with the family, or great moments in their life, or even the little things of the day. They always seem cheerful. These same people see the unfortunate incidents of their lives in the third person. They can remember past incidents and themselves as participants, but without having to re-live the emotional state of that time. On the other hand, people who are depressed and unhappy do the opposite; they see the positive things in the third person (as though they had not actually been there at the time and shared in the joy); and they see negative things in the first person, re-living the distress. Keeping focussed on their problems takes most of their attention so their lives seem flat and dull.[10] Two other ways to remember are: remembering all events in the first person, which makes for a continual roller-coaster ride, or remembering all events in the third person, which makes for a very even-tempered life.

Intriguingly, we can learn to have some control over the degree of emotion that we re-experience when we remember a particular incident from the past. This type of control is like the control we have over breathing. If we don't pay attention to it, our breathing is automatic, speeding up when we do exercise and slowing down when we rest. If we don't think about it, the memories of our past are seen in first or third person depending on how the system has previously retrieved those memories. However, if we choose to, it is possible to switch between seeing the action through the eyes of the central player, to seeing it as a neutral observer.

> *Events in themselves are neither good nor bad. We judge the events in our lives, colouring them with our own perceptions. The perception affects our memory of the event … in this exercise you are not changing the event, you're changing your perception of the event.*[11]

Occasionally the emotion in an unwanted memory will be neutralised just by switching perspective, but often further work is required. Emotions attached to an event can be revised by mentally reviewing your interpretation – 'the script', as it is sometimes called. You can change the memory to something small, dull and distant, with yourself as you are now as a neutral observer. To disarm a memory in this way:

- Find somewhere you feel safe, comfortable and in control.

- Think of the event.

- Dissociate from it by moving out of your body to see it happening far away from you.

- Imagine looking at the incident through a thick dull glass.

- See it in boring colours – greys and dull browns.

- Make the image smaller and further away from yourself.

- Say out loud 'That person over there was embarrassed/frightened /unhappy' (whichever is appropriate), knowing 'that person' was a younger version of yourself at another time.

This technique replaces the personal with the impersonal, makes a statement about it in the past tense and paves the way for diminishing the strength of the emotions. Although the process alters none of the facts of what happened, and may not prevent a memory from surfacing, for some people it is an effective technique to detach the emotional impact of the memory.[12]

A different method of down-playing an incident is described by Anthony Robbins. He makes a parody of it by imagining he is making a home movie of the incident:

Imagine the old pattern as a movie. Play it forwards fast, and then backwards, a dozen times. Scramble the images, change colours and speed, put ridiculous Mickey Mouse hats on the bad guys, and make yourself large and strong, to break the pattern. As we change the images, we change how we feel.[13]

Try the techniques that work for you

There is no one answer that addresses all problems with recurring unpleasant memories. The brain has such extraordinary retentive abilities that happening upon the right set of cues will reactivate a long past memory. One can't help that. What one can help is the emotional importance given to the matter. There is much variation in how different people respond to the different techniques. Try the ones that appeal.

Persistent traumatic memories[14]

Persistent traumatic memories can be of life-threatening situations like accidents or war, sexual abuse, the onset of serious illness, or the death of a loved one. It is estimated that 50 per cent of people will suffer from a traumatic experience sometime in their lives. In occupations like ambulance work, fire fighting and rescue work, everyday duties can leave the workers with horrifying flashbacks that can recur for weeks.

There is ongoing debate in the memory literature about whether fearful and disturbing memories are encoded, stored and remembered by the same mechanisms as all other memories.[15] What is clear is that a memory persists because of the strength of the emotion attached to it, and in traumatic memories the emotion is very strong. In extreme cases a person can feel all the physical symptoms of intense fear – sweaty palms and pumping heart – just by remembering a long-past fearful incident. Psychologist Daniel Schacter notes that people are not just remembering the past event, they are reliving it.[16] How long painful memories continue to disturb people after an event depends on how they have dealt with those memories.

> *… long-lasting persistence is not an inevitable consequence of all disappointments: how we respond to adversity, and whether we become plagued by persistence, depends on how we evaluate and appraise what happens to us.'*[17]

Schacter suggests that we need to learn to live with memory's power, neither actively suppressing the memory, nor continually ruminating on it.

He considers that 'for the long-term, confronting, disclosing and integrating those experiences we would most like to forget is the most effective counter to persistence'.[18]

Talking through the event with a good friend or therapist is helpful. Since the brain can't help recalling the event, to do so in a safe environment helps in the habituation process, the lessening of the physical impact of the troublesome memories and the natural grieving process.

Learning new technology

How to tackle it; how not to be worried by it.
WENDY

Many people are intimidated by technology such as programming video players and mistakenly think it is hard because they are getting older. The fact is that 95 per cent of the population have a video player and only a fraction know how to program it. The fault is in poor design of the appliance, or the instructions or both.

The easiest information to recall is something that is already very familiar, or that we have recalled recently. If we are learning something quite strange to us, like new technology, it is important to find some point of familiarity that can be used as the entrance point to the new learning. People say 'I just couldn't get a handle on it' when describing the feeling of not being able to fit new information in with what they already know. One good way of tackling something complicated is to break it down into smaller segments, but if the technology is unfamiliar we often don't know what the components are.

What's the difference between technology that we can cope with, like telephones, fridges and washing machines, and those appliances that we feel just aren't worth the trouble of mastering? Roger Schanks suggests that doing something like using a telephone can be described as a story that has a sequence of actions.[19] You pick up the handset, listen for the dial tone, dial the number, hold the handpiece to your ear, and say hello when the other end answers. It's actually quite a complicated sequence of actions, but we have been doing it for years and it's familiar. If a change fits into the 'story', such as a new kind of handset, we accommodate quickly, but if the story changes, such as a machine answering instead of a person and starts telling us to press 1 for this and 2 for that, we need to rewrite the script of the story to understand how it works.

Technology can get a lot more complicated than telephones; for example, the instructions for computers are often incomprehensible. So many instruction manuals are badly written because they assume we already know the buzz words and the 'story'.

As well as inventing its own jargon, new technology appropriates perfectly good everyday words and gives them additional meanings. The words in an explanation may appear familiar: for example, using the term 'viruses' to refer to rogue programs that are not meant to be on a computer. But familiarity is wearing a false face. People new to computers used to cringe away from a machine if they were told that it had a virus. That word was part of the story that described ills of the human body, but this virus can't be caught by humans. Now the word must be shared with computer ailments.

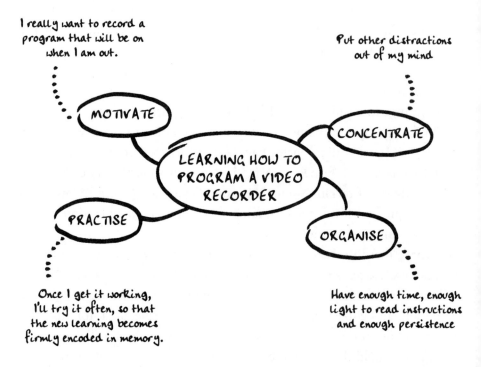

A concept map showing how the four steps of learning something new can be applied to learning to program a video recorder. Begin with the four steps of motivate, concentrate, organise and practice and then expand on each of these as shown.

To learn new technology:

- Don't worry so much about breaking the appliance that you can't get started.

- Start with the knowledge that it's going to be different.

- Make sure you can clearly see all its fiddly bits.

- Find points of similarity between old and new – get a grasp of its 'story'.

- Play with it, spend time with the new, mess around with it, so that its strangeness grows into familiarity.

- Read the manual as though some words were in a foreign language that you need to translate (highlight the unfamiliar ones and seek explanations from the manufacturer's customer service).

- Write down what you have to do or underline the steps in the manual.

- Use what you have learned.

- Learn small amounts at a time, continually going back and revising earlier items.

A statistics lecturer once described the introductory process as 'getting your hands dirty with it'. The people who adapt to new technology really well don't treat it as a serious business, they treat it as fun.

Remembering numbers in everyday life

Do we build in blocks to recall by self-talk, e.g. saying things like 'I have a bad memory', 'I can never remember names/numbers'?
ANITA

Many Memory Survey respondents mentioned difficulty with remembering numbers. In answer to Anita's question, negative self-talk can affect our willingness to concentrate and practise numbers, but the problem is not just our own attitude. There are so many numbers to remember in this increasingly numbered world – phone numbers, postcodes, numberplates, and PIN numbers for credit cards – to name some of the common ones.

Phone numbers are frequently said too quickly to hear properly, and on answer machines they are often gabbled so quickly that it is not possible to write them down. Often one needs to listen to a phone message three times, writing down a few more digits each time. The problem arises because people can talk much faster than they can listen and comprehend. Phone numbers said in pairs and rhythmically are much easier to hear and remember (at least for long enough to write down).

oh-one	nine-two	six-five	five-oh
0-1	9-2	6-5	5-0

Identification numbers were developed for the convenience of machines, not people. Mathematically minded people find patterns in numbers and regard them as old friends, but for most of us it makes sense to write down the secret ones for credit cards and store them somewhere safe. There are just a few numbers very useful to know, like the numberplate of a car and a special phone number. It is worthwhile finding a scheme to remember them. For these, good strategies involve word games, pictures and patterns.

Numbers at our fingertips

Many people remember sequences of key presses for phone numbers or automatic teller machines 'in their fingertips'. Our brains are specialised to understand how to move around in space, and turning sequences of numbers into finger movements is very effective.

A particular PIN is like a sequence of directions over the keypad on an automatic teller. For example, 1-3-7-4 starts in the top left corner, jumps to the right, then diagonally left, and finally halfway back up. It sounds clumsy in words, but when we trace it out with our fingers, it is tracing a triangle and easy to remember.

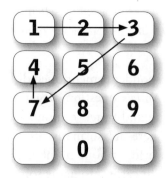

Memory in our fingertips for the PIN 1374.

Words, rhymes and mini-stories

> *When my grandmother bought her fruit and veg in her little country town, the greengrocer would carry the box back to the car for her as she continued on with her shopping. He needed to know the numberplate – CHP164 – but my grandmother had a lot of trouble with numbers so she invented a little story: 'Come Here Pup, one sick paw.' For me, growing up a city kid, that mnemonic symbolised my grandmother's inventiveness, her kindness and her life as a country woman. It's now 30 years later and I still remember my grandmother's numberplate. I don't think I could ever forget it.*
>
> LANA (A FRIEND)

When our memory system blocks on numbers, the problem is often just getting started. For example, to remember the numberplate VTR123, a mnemonic for the first three letters could be 'VTR: very tough retiree', and once the letters are started the numbers will just roll on.

> *[I regret] being unable to instantly remember (as previously) when asked my home telephone number.*
>
> CON

As with car numberplates, the strategy for phone numbers is to find a mnemonic for the beginning of the number sequence and the rest of it follows. A friend, Lynda, remembers an eight-digit phone number as a whimsical look at her own life at four different ages:

01 age at which I took my first step
92 age at which I will climb Mt Everest
65 age at which I will retire
50 age at which I would like to retire

A colleague has for years used a system for remembering up to four numbers by involving the members of her family and mealtimes. For example, for the number 1736, she visualises the kitchen of her house when the children were frenetic teenagers, and thinks, 'One child for dinner at 7 and the other three at 6', which shortens to '1 (for) 7 (and) 3 (for) 6.'

Asking around your friends can reveal a quite ingenious array of systems for remembering numbers. The important part is for people to find something significant or amusing to themselves.

Numbers as patterns

For phone numbers I use patterns but then I have been a maths teacher all my life.
BRIDGET

Some people like numbers and see them as friends. The number 247 may be special because it is their numberplate. The number 25 might be easy to remember because that's the age they were when they were married. The number 527 could be remembered as 5+2 = 7. Some people imagine their phone number as stairs – very irregular stairs!

We know of one retired mathematician who had heart surgery and had to be awake and calm during the operation. He spent the time thinking about numbers and calculated that his hospital bed number, 917776, was exactly equal to 304 x 3019. No doubt he can still remember or reconstruct that number!

To people who like numbers, they are not just meaningless symbols, strung together arbitrarily. Sequences of numbers can form patterns, just like sequences of letters can form words. There are so many ways that numbers can form patterns that it becomes a game, and some aid to memory can almost always be found.

Methods of the masters

People with memory abilities beyond the normal range show us just how much the human mind can achieve. Do they have special brains or are their skills due to practice (or obsession)? Just as there are variations in abilities within the normal range, there is a wide range outside the norm. Some skills are acquired through hard work, others through unusual talents.

Linking ideas to locations – method of loci

Who is that man moving slowly in the lonely building, stopping at intervals with an intent face? He is a rhetoric student forming a set of memory loci.[20]

The ancient Greek and Roman orators remembered their speeches with astonishing accuracy by using a mnemonic strategy called the 'method of loci'. They composed their lengthy speeches by moving from place to place in noble lofty buildings. The Roman master orator and writer Cicero suggested:

> *Assign to them exceptional beauty or singular ugliness; … or if we somehow disfigure them, as by introducing one stained with blood or soiled with mud … or by assigning certain comic effects to our images … that too will ensure our remembering them more readily.*[21]

The association of one idea to one physical place relieves the orator of having to remember a lot of items all at once. Since it is a sequence, one place-plus-thought calls up the next place-plus-thought. Unless rehearsed, the ideas attached to the special places will fade, leaving the sites free for the next set of items.

The method of loci is an inspiring example from the glory days of oratory. With proper preparation it effectively encodes and stores the material and provides effective recall cues to remember long sequences. We don't know anyone who practises this method in everyday use. (It works, but it's quicker and easier to use notes.) Francis Yates makes the same point even more forcefully: 'There is no doubt that the method will work for anyone who is prepared to labour seriously at these mnemonic gymnastics.'[22]

Turning numbers into pictures – the peg method

Many people have heard of the peg method which is used by several professional mnemonists to remember sequences of numbers. It is based on the idea of turning numbers into words, and then combining the words to form pictures. First, one needs to learn ten picture-number pairs for the numbers zero to nine, such as one is a bun, two is a shoe, three is a tree etc.

Then, to remember a two digit number, create an image combining the two corresponding pictures. For example, to remember 23, turn 2 into shoe and 3 into tree, and then picture a shoe-tree (a new species!).

Several commercial audio tapes that claim to improve memory teach the peg method. It requires a fair bit of effort to learn, and good visualisation skills to apply, and is undoubtedly effective for those who master the technique and keep practising. Intrigued with how frequently such mnemonics are actually used in everyday life, we asked around and found that even when people had done a course and thoroughly learned the method, the longest time they actually used it varied from a few days up to a year.

> *I can still remember the mnemonics I used 35 years ago but have difficulty in recalling what they stand for.*
> HELENA

We mention the peg method since so many people have heard of it or similar systems, but we doubt that it is easy or practical enough for everyday memory lapses. Its saving grace is that it is fun to learn, and for anyone interested in the method there is plenty of good detailed published material.[23]

> *Vether it's worthwhile goin' through so much to learn so little, as the charity-boy said ven he got to the end of the alphabet, is a matter of taste.*
> CHARLES DICKENS[24]

Super memories of the memory gifted

It might seem unfortunate that our memory systems do not remember everything we want them to, but would we really want to remember every trifling item our eyes chanced to light upon, every name read or heard? Every number? One person who almost did just that was an amazing man named Shereshevski. He remembered practically everything. The distinguished Russian linguist and psychologist Aleksandr Luria described his own amazement when he could not devise exacting enough tests to probe the depths of Shereshevski's memory.[25] Lists of more than 100 digits, poetry in unknown languages, or scientific formulae were promptly reproduced even many years later.

These astounding memory abilities came from Shereshevski's innate ability to match words, even nonsense words, with images. To remember a huge list of names or numbers (which his brain treated in the same way) he needed a few seconds after hearing each item while he imagined it positioned in a certain place such as against a fence. When asked to recall the list, even 15 years later, he would mentally walk along the fence and 'see' each item. On the few occasions that he missed one, he simply did not 'see' an upright pencil against the upright posts of the fence, or a white egg against a white fence.

His super-normal memory was not without difficulties in everyday life. Relentlessly and unceasingly, every sound he heard – words, numbers, people coughing, even changes in tone when someone was speaking – would call up colours and images. This linking of the senses is called synesthesia. His unusual memory caused him difficulty in daily functioning and confusion in understanding the meaning of abstract thoughts and ideas.

Chess and bridge

I am a keen bridge player and strangely I never forget
a card played or the number of cards played.
GISLA

It is estimated that chess masters know 50,000 chess games, but not by rote memory. What they know is the integral relationship between all the pieces in a very large number of games. Chess masters have superior powers of organisation and see a chessboard as an integrated whole, not just individual pieces. Similarly, bridge players can have phenomenal memories for games and can recall every card from games that were played even years earlier. It might seem that bridge and chess masters would have special brains in some way like Shereshevski, but interestingly they generally have ordinary memories for ordinary life. Their special skills in their own fields reflect the depth and richness that comes from long experience, intense involvement and huge effort.

Memory competitions

Outstanding performance in the mnemonic, athletic and musical
fields … is always associated with huge amounts of practice – the
perspiration rather than the inspiration theory of genius.[26]

In memory competitions, competitors are timed while they memorise a full pack of cards in any order, pages of faces and names, train timetables, achievements of athletes, or thousands of numbers and words. However, such abilities don't come without effort. Those who take on challenges like national and world memory competitions achieve their outstanding feats of memory with huge amounts of practice.

Paradoxically, the 1999 winner of the USA National Memory Championship was incredibly absentminded and relied on sticky notes to do her shopping![27] One would have thought that she could employ the super-effective techniques of competition winning to conduct her daily life, but perhaps it was not worth the effort. The achievements of the masters leaves us feeling awed and astonished, so it's something of a relief to note at least one of them uses a list when going shopping.

The brain gets better at the things it does often. Different regions of the brain are specialised to take care of different facets of memory, so knowledge of where to put effort can be used to maximise results. 'Memory' is too complex a property to be 'improved' across the board in a global sweep. Like getting fit, it needs selective training and a bit at a time.

> *Memory is better the more we have a reason to study, the more we like what we are studying, and the more we can bring the full breadth of our personality to the moment of learning.*[28]

At a glance

- Good organisational systems make things 'easy to file and easy to find'. They are styled to suit the person who needs to use them.

- Working memory capacity can be boosted for big tasks like moving house by using lists and concept maps.

- Improving memory in social situations involves practising names and anecdotes before events, mentally rehearsing during the events and reviewing the names, and gracefully sliding over 'senior's moments'.

- It is probably not possible to completely forget unwanted memories but they can be made less intrusive by changing one's perspective on them.

- Persistent traumatic memories can be dealt with over time by using the techniques of confronting, disclosing and integrating.

- To learn new technology, begin at some point of familiarity; understand the 'story'; spend time with it to ease its strangeness; interpret the manual as though it were in a foreign language.

- To hear and remember phone numbers, the digits should be said in pairs and rhythmically.

- To remember PINS and other number sequences, find rhythm and patterns in them, or turn them into stories.

- Some phenomenal memory abilities are acquired through exceptional practice and others are sheer genius.

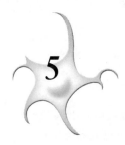

Normal Ageing and Normal Forgetting

Nature gives to every time and season
some beauties of its own.
Charles Dickens[1]

In today's society there is general agreement about appropriate times for the progressive stages of social life. Young people are expected to move from relying on support from their parents to earning their own living. Older people are expected to retire from full-time work, then gradually disengage from former activities and become forgetful. Is it inevitable they 'lose their memories'? There is certainly a general perception that this is so! But for the majority of longer-living, healthier, older people, core memory is preserved, although it is normal for memory to slow down a bit and for its owner to be more conscious of memory lapses.

Memory is essential in the maintenance of our normal daily lives. It contains our sense of identity stemming from our past and it carries our hopes and plans for the future. Small wonder that we worry if we think our memories are disappearing. Ironically, worry itself, even about memory loss, can make that loss temporarily worse. Since memory is so important in our lives, it ranks high as a subject of study. Researchers have found that some aspects of memory do deteriorate in older people (and we have found agreement between these findings and our own Memory Survey). In this chapter we aim to alleviate anxiety about memory lapses by describing normal changes in memory abilities specifically due to age (rather than disease), why this happens and what can be done about it.

Concepts of normality

What is normal – because with increased age
you are more conscious of memory loss.
Leonie

The concept of normal growth has been studied extensively. What is 'normal' is established by charting what 75 per cent of healthy individuals do in the sequence of life's milestones. The term 'milestone' dates back to when we measured distance in miles, and there actually were white painted stones by the roadside that gave the distance from the last town. They let you know how you were getting on. Life also has its milestones.

The concept of normality includes individual variation in timing when each milestone is reached. For example, one child might read at six years and another at seven years – both are within the normal range. Researchers who study brain and body functioning in older adults are discovering a similar range of normality in later life. Life span developmentalists are interested in changes over the entire life span, with the purpose of optimising the functioning of both mind and body.[2]

In the past, all old people were expected to develop dementia. In fact dementia was equated with old age, but the development of better diagnostic tools during the 1990s has allowed a much more scientific appraisal of memory. Memory loss is associated with some loss of brain cells in certain regions of the brain. There is now scientific acknowledgment of normal, mild, brain decline, referred to by memory researchers as 'age-associated memory impairments'. By contrast, memory impairments caused by diseases of the brain are not normal. The differences between memory lapses due to normal ageing and the early stages of dementia diseases such as Alzheimer's are discussed fully in Chapter 6, 'Normal Memory Loss or Alzheimer's?'.

Researchers refer to our capacity for memory, intelligence, reasoning and understanding as 'cognition', which are controlled from different parts of the brain. Memory is only one component. The small losses of memory function discussed below do not mean that the other aspects of cognition are lost too. Difficulty with names and words is part of the normal slowing down of memory with ageing, rather like greying of hair. The owners might regret the greying but it need not disrupt independent living.

Is it normal to forget?

It would be interesting to find out that these are just common lapses due to ageing and not something more serious.
TARA

Yes, it is normal to forget some things, and no, it is not normal for memory loss to seriously disrupt everyday life. In normal ageing most people do have some memory lapses where a desired name or word won't come quickly to mind. The table below lists those aspects of memory that generally stay good with age and those that can worsen with age.

Aspects of memory[3]	
Mostly endure with age	Can worsen with age
• Knowledge about people and things (semantic mmory)	• Tip-of-tongue occurrences
• Remembering the gist of long-ago events	• Remembering with no prompt (self-initiated recall)
• A strong sense of self and emotional maturity	• Future intentions if no reminder cues
• Learning and using reminder strategies	• Juggling more than one thing at a time
• Remembering well if more time taken	• Remembering under time pressure
• Remembering if given cue	• The source of information (episodic memory)

• Skills already learned (existing procedural memory)	• Stopping the wrong word from slipping out
• Using implicit memory, especially priming	• Learning new physical skills (new procedural memory)

Eight aspects of memory that mostly endure with age

The following aspects of memory generally stay good with age because they do not place much demand on attention.[4]

KNOWLEDGE ABOUT PEOPLE AND THINGS

> *[Are] lapses due to having to remember and recall more information as one ages?*
> **VERONICA**

Our vast store of general knowledge (semantic memory) stays good with age. We are not likely to forget that the moon orbits the earth, though few people would remember when they learned that fact. The semantic memory system includes the knowledge of how to do things like catch a train, banking, telephoning, housekeeping and using common sense, which is probably a long accumulation of skills and coping strategies.[5] It is also used to make inferences and solve problems.

Does the memory system fill up? Certainly a person encounters more information through having lived a long time, but in semantic memory there would be innumerable links between items and concepts. Such a network makes recall easier, not harder, and there is plenty of room in the brain for the expansion of networks. Over the years, single ideas become a collection of interrelated ideas, personalised to each individual. A linked network is created which allows easy recall of any one of the items. As we age, our store of knowledge – semantic memory – continues to grow into a vast, interconnected net of ideas and inferences. That knowledge (once called wisdom) is far more than information, and is reflected in the fact that traditional folklore often associated youth with impatience and age with wisdom.

Remembering the gist of long-ago events

We can forget the details, and we can therefore form concepts and gradually absorb knowledge by adding up the lessons from different kinds of experiences ... some degree of forgetting, as it occurs in healthy individuals, is an important and necessary part of normal memory function.[6]

Just as remembering the gist of a sentence is easier than remembering the exact words, so also remembering the gist of an event is easier than recalling the exact details. The memory lets go of items that are not of critical importance.

Details from long-past events in our lives are often only generated as probable events, consistent with main themes. If details are important, the key to more accurate remembering is to use very specific cues such as old photographs or letters.

Strong sense of self and emotional maturity

The best prediction about how the years will change us is that they will not.[7]

In normal ageing our sense of who we are is undiminished. Our accumulation of memories from the past supports our sense of self, knowledge of where we have been and what we have done. Over the years we build our identities from the 'I' feeling within us. Semantic memory includes the sense of self – one's own personality and life skills. Different generations can have differing world views because of events of the times, but individual personalities remain stable.[8]

Learning and using reminder strategies

Is it possible that a reliable system may evolve whereby we old people, still coherent and alert, could improve the memory loss?
Felicity

Older people who are coherent and alert can improve memory loss. Training improves whichever system is specifically targeted by the mental exercise, as the following study showed.

Starting with the premise that cognitive training improves memory, researcher Steve Zarit and his colleagues gave cognitive training to one group of volunteer older people, and discussion sessions to a second group.[9] Both groups believed that their memories would be helped. The researchers found that complaints about memory lessened in both groups, but objective testing showed that only in the group receiving the training in use of strategies did memory actually improve. This result is very interesting on two counts: first, that direct teaching of strategies really does work; and second, the positive effect on morale. Believing that they were being helped removed many of the complaints about memory of the control group, even though their memory abilities remained the same as before the discussion sessions. If we think we have no need to worry, the actual memory loss seems not to be a problem.

The study also found that older people tended to use the same strategies all the time even when they were ineffective. However, they could learn new strategies when shown how to do this by direct teaching. Participants were taught to use imaginative aids: for example, to remember the time of a 12 o'clock appointment by imagining someone waiting for a friend with two arms held straight above their head, like the two arms of a clock. We have described similar strategies in earlier chapters.

Older people need three extra considerations to learn new strategies: remove time constraints, keep the learning relevant to older people, and if new material must be learned, begin at some point of familiarity to them.[10]

REMEMBERING WELL IF MORE TIME TAKEN

Taking longer to do things and think of things is difficult in an age that wants instant everything, from coffee to computers. When we age, the memory systems work the same but we take more time about it. Older people can do as well as younger people if given more time.[11]

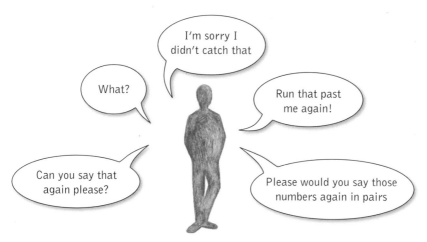

If you need more time, ask for it!

Remembering if given cue

The question, 'Is her name Mary?' is much easier to answer than 'What's her name?' The two questions show the difference between recognition (which stays good with age) and free recall (which is more difficult and gets harder with age). Remembering when given partial hints (cued recall) is intermediate in difficulty between these two. The more cues we are given, the easier is the task of remembering.

Scrutinising memory takes more time and effort as we age. For example, if a reminder invoice indicates that a bill is overdue we may have been sure it had been paid. The cheque butt shows it has been written, but was it really posted? When accurate memory of an event is required, Daniel Schacter advocates a rule of thumb to always demand from one's memory recollections of distinctive details of an experience.[12] Scrutinising memory means searching for mental details of the how, when and where it was posted. These confirming details are absent if the posting had been merely an intention.

Skills already learned

The procedural memory system (also part of the implicit memory system) remembers how to do physical things. Possibly the skills were learned many years ago, like typing, riding a bike or playing a musical instrument. Muscles might get out of condition but the mind does not forget what should be done. This story from a friend, Louise, illustrates the point: 'When my friend Macquarie turned 75 he had to do a driving test to renew his driving licence and his grandson was trying for his first licence. The same examiner tested them both on a route with a one-way street. Macquarie, with his years of driving experience, passed with flying colours and much congratulation. The 18 year old also passed, since his handling of the car was good, but with advice to think ahead next time he drove into a one-way street.'

Intertwined with procedural memory in a driving test is semantic memory, which is needed to remember road rules and understand the implications of the term 'one-way street' when driving.[13] Reflexes may be slower as we age, but both knowledge of the road rules and how to drive the car remain good.

> *As we are going to visit some people I ask my wife their name and I repeat it while we reach their place.*
> **CARLOS**

The implicit memory system (that part which is below our level of awareness) includes priming, which is the influence of recent events upon memory and of which we are not necessarily conscious. As we described in Chapter 3, to be able to recall names quickly, review them up to 24 hours before the event. Similarly, if there is a problem or something to sort out, it helps to have a look at it and then give the non-conscious memory a chance to quietly sort out ideas and priorities. These are all part of the well-preserved implicit memory system. Priming for implicit memory does not suffer with age because it does not need the self-initiated, deliberate search as does explicit memory.[15]

Eight aspects of memory that can worsen with age

> *When the problem of remembering first becomes apparent, our reaction seems to be a feeling of anger and resentment but worse, that we are getting old!*
> **FELICITY**

The following aspects of memory can become worse with age.

TIP-OF-TONGUE OCCURANCES

The most common complaint of older people is the frustrating phenomenon called tip-of-tongue.[16] When a familiar name won't surface, it is not that the memory doesn't have the name tucked away somewhere, it's just that it won't surface at the right moment. This phenomenon happens at all ages, but more so for older people.

REMEMBERING WITH NO PROMPT

> *[It's a problem] forgetting key words when talking to doctors.*
> **SUZETTE**

Remembering 'cold turkey' is difficult for older brains. Self-initiated retrieval cues are more difficult with ageing since the links must be found from within one's own memory. The difficulty is reduced if a relevant context is provided. For example, recalling the name of someone who lives in your street is easier if you meet them in your street rather than somewhere entirely different.

Difficulties with spontaneous recall don't mean that the memory is not in there. It may have needed a stronger encoding, more time to surface, or the original setting to activate the right prompts.

When visiting a doctor, many people find they have three or four things to ask about. It is usually easy to remember the first thing to ask about, but the answer might drive the other questions out of one's mind. It is quite reasonable to take a list of items as a reminder of the questions to be asked. It is also easy to forget the answers. Writing down the doctor's answers to each question ensures future remembering. Taking a written list of current medications to present to doctors is also a good idea.

FUTURE INTENTIONS IF NO REMINDER CUES[17]

> *[I forget] to do things, e.g. buy a paper on the way home.*
> **MEREDITH**

Older people have more difficulty remembering to do something at a future time (prospective memory). Both types of prospective memory, time-based (e.g. phone at 10 am) and event-based (e.g. phone when you get home) are liable to be forgotten unless effective physical cues can be set up.[18] However, older people can use tangible reminders very effectively.

JUGGLING MORE THAN ONE THING AT A TIME

> *I find the lack of ability to handle/consider multiple tasks and decisions at one time a real worry. The 'I can cope with only one thing at a time' is becoming very frustrating. When I was younger, handling multi-tasks was so routine.*
> **ELVIRA**

Working memory is needed when trying to do two things at once and there are competing demands for attention. This could happen if you are interrupted while looking after children or there are too many distractions while driving a car. Situations that require juggling several essential items can overload working memory capacity.

Working memory is one system that is often less effective as we age because it is dependent on keeping one's attention on several things at once.[19] For maximum efficiency, concentrate on one thing at a time, alternating if there are competing demands.

REMEMBERING UNDER TIME PRESSURE

> *The problem of arriving at an intersection and can't think quickly enough as to which is the fastest way to go – left or right!*
> **CON**

Older people make more mistakes if they are required to hurry. They function much better if they are given extra time to think about something. In the story of Macquarie and his grandson, if the driving examiner told both applicants that they were to make a right-hand turn at the end of a one-way street, thus giving them both time and opportunity to think ahead and move into the appropriate lane, the early notice could be used to advantage by the older man. Had something quite unexpected happened that required instant braking, one would expect the reaction time of the young man to be much quicker.

THE SOURCE OF INFORMATION

Although tip-of-tongue is the most common memory complaint of older people, there are actually larger deficits in forming new episodic memories. Older people have less ability to consciously recall exactly when and where something happened, for example, telling a joke back to the friend who told it to you. As we get older, the source of information learned even last week can become more difficult to place.

STOPPING THE WRONG WORD FROM SLIPPING OUT

> *I wonder how much one's memory lapses can be attributed to failing ~~conversation~~ concentration (the mistake in this line is an example!).*
> **GERALDINE**

Writing 'conversation' instead of 'concentration' happens because of the brain's failure to inhibit the wrong word. Word substitutes like this often have the same characteristics as the intended word, such as beginning with the same letter and being about the same length. The substitute may be a more common word and often slips out towards the end of a sentence when your attention has moved on to something else. However, these small stumbles are not serious and just show that there is some slackening off in one of the language areas of the brain.

Older people can be more distracted by irrelevant thoughts and events, like personal memories inadvertently called up by what they were saying or something else going on at the same time. The distractions result from less efficient inhibitory processes. There is a tendency to shy away from the more difficult task of searching memory for the intended word or fact and to instead seize on the word or thought most easily accessible.

Learning new physical skills

It will come as no surprise that learning a new physical skill (new procedural memory) is harder for older people. For example, we can learn a game like croquet but it does get harder for mind and muscles to learn to work together.

*   *   *

> *God grant me the senility to forget the people I never liked anyway, the good fortune to run into the ones that I do, and the eyesight to tell the difference.*
> ANON

Memory for long ago

> *Last year I went back to my home town for 3 weeks, after an absence of 50 years, during which my contact had only been through the gossip in the letters of relatives. I was quite amazed at how the distant past comes back in detail – conversations, relationships, details of houses and landforms, classmates' names (many of them now dead).*
> GERALDINE

Many of the Memory Survey respondents enthusiastically reported incidents from the past and marvelled that memory for long ago should be so clear while recent memory was so uncertain. Some also described the trigger (the cue) that brought the memory to mind.

For example, when revisiting your old home town and seeing people once well known, floods of memories come back because of the multitude and specificity of the cues. If you talk about your cousin Jack, that's slightly stimulating your memory recall. If Jack actually walks through the door he embodies a dozen cues. You see his smile and all his features, hear his voice, touch his hand, remember again the way he walks.

Survey respondents emphasised the vividness of memories from childhood, but there are likely to be many more memories that are not recalled, which lack the vividness and excitement of losses and celebrations. Perhaps they were not firmly encoded, or were encoded at the time but faded with lack of recall, or blurred into similar memories.

General gist rather than detail[20]

> I recently told a friend that I had a very distinctive childhood memory of watching Judy Garland sing 'Somewhere over the Rainbow' from within a white moon in the movie The Wizard of Oz when I was aged 3 years. Recently, we looked at a video of the movie and my rehearsed memory had joined two things in the movie, but she was not in the moon.
>
> CHRIS

It is very difficult to believe that one could be mistaken when a visual image is very strong, but in fact vividness is not necessarily a measure of accurate recall of details. Graphic memory is more of a comment on how our memories work than a measure of reality. We all have favourite memories of some happy event and ones that show us in a favourable light, and we strengthen them by thinking of them often. Like a car or favourite shoes that you polish often, vividness in memory is polished with every recall. People are especially prone to forget how much a memory has been polished. Often we remember the general gist of a long past event but the details have become merged or simplified. We have no way of knowing if this is the case unless there is proof. The Wizard of Oz was a wonderful children's film, full of magical happenings, so it would be entirely consistent with the general tenor of the film to show the actress singing from the moon, but which she did not actually do.

As Larry Squire and Eric Kandel explain, '... forgetting is an important part of remembering. People need to forget or pass over the details in order to grasp the gist and they need to set aside the details in order to appreciate similarity and metaphor and to form general concepts.'[21] Feelings and small details about an event can also subtly change with each remembering. We can be influenced by the comments of others, or even just with the passage of time and the many later experiences we have had.

Memories become individualised to each person

I have found that episodes that appeared important in my life were totally forgotten by my children. They usually had their own memories of the past.

HANNAH

The predominance of generalised perspective over detail also contributes to differences between people's recall of the same event. We own our experiences in our own individual way. The mix includes how we felt at the time and the importance of the event in our life.

Another reason for differing versions is the personality of an individual. One may have a 'big picture' view of the world and be impatient of details (particularly if they spoil a good story), another person might find satisfaction in ferreting out details. We can only remember what we have encoded. What we notice and encode strongly depends on who we are and what is meaningful to us at the time.[22]

Patricia Hampl suggests that the best way to discover what you feel about the past is to write your life story, and that the real job of memoir is to seek congruence between memories and their hidden emotions.[23] Hampl goes on to say that perspective combines with memory facts to give meaning and ownership to past experience. Everyone needs to have a good opinion of themselves and subtle changes in remembered details of long ago can help achieve this satisfactory account. In the working over of long-ago memories, and in sharing those intimacies with others, we maintain psychological and emotional well-being.[24] This view of memory emphasises the recall of long-ago memories as necessary reconstructions in order to live comfortably in the present.

A strong sense of self

Identity is explored during adolescence as a teenager seeks answers to such questions as 'Who am I?' and 'What do I believe in?' The answers can veer around wildly for a number of years, but usually by the late twenties the person has established an identity, a set of beliefs, some of which become core values. In general, goals throughout life become less idealistic and more achievable.[25]

Musing over the past clarifies one's own strong sense of self and where one belongs in the general scheme of things. Collecting and sharing with family and friends the fabric of earlier times is particularly important for people who have left their homeland to settle somewhere else. There is a need to preserve family identities by passing on memories of all sorts of little anecdotes and traditions. To keep our sense of identity robust, we need to keep the significance of an event, as well as its occurrence. The significance is what the event meant in our lives both then and now. Where families are separated, memories can be preserved in photographs and in the written word. Family ties are strengthened by the sharing and working over of collective memories.

> For the past eighty years I have started each day in the same manner. It is not a mechanical routine but something essential to my daily life. I go to the piano, and I play two preludes and fugues of Bach. I cannot think of doing otherwise. It is a sort of benediction on the house. But that is not its only meaning for me. It is a rediscovery of the world of which I have the joy of being a part. It fills me with awareness of the wonder of life, with a feeling of the incredible marvel of being a human being.
> PABLO CASALS (THEN AGED 93)[26]

Differences between older and younger people

> Something I must remark on is the proportion of younger friends, e.g. in forties and fifties, who say, 'Oh, that happens to me. I have a hopeless memory'. I wonder if this is becoming more prevalent or are they just trying to comfort me?
> GERALDINE

Some differences between the memory powers at younger and older ages become noticeable around the age of 60, although the slow decline may have begun at least 20 years or more before that. (To be quite precise, ageing begins at conception.) Memory powers are thought to peak in the early twenties with some fluctuations and some loss each decade from then on. Small memory losses from middle age onwards are normal. Of course, in normal ageing it does not dwindle to nothing.[27] In every age group there are large variations among individuals.

> Have always been a bit vague about people's names. In a way am a little better than when young in this respect being more aware of

*my failing. Think it is best to keep calm, take notes as reminders
and cope with each day's problems as they crop up.*
CLAUDE

The fact is that some people forget names and some people are good at
remembering names, regardless of age. The good ones pay a lot of attention
to names and review them, and of course they reinforce themselves by
knowing they are good. Others do not – and possibly never have – attended
in detail to the names of those around them. Still others do not let the little
lapses bother them. We heard of one lady who had a lapse while giving a
speech at a wedding, and covered the slight delay with great poise, saying
'Ah, I just had a senior's moment!'

The Third and Fourth Ages

The period of life often called the Third Age (usually considered to be
60 to 85 years) is a social and biological distinction, based on the usual
retirement age and the tendency of the body to slow down a bit. There is
increasing recognition of a Fourth Age beginning at age 85 which differs in
many ways from the Third Age. A study of over 80 year olds suggested that
those who live to old-old ages have resilience and coping strategies to deal
with life's ups and downs, sometimes referred to as a 'hardy survivor' effect.
An interesting observation from the study was that a person's expectation
of life might be more important than whether the events of their life were
desirable or undesirable.[28] Other studies have also found links between
positive attitudes to ageing and survival (see further details in Chapter 7,
'Maintaining Health for Vintage Memories').[29] In an ABC Radio interview
on centenarians, Norman Swan asked: 'The key question for those people
who would like to live to 100 is, is it simply writ in your genes?'[30] The answer
from Tom Perls of Harvard Medical School was that 'most people have genes
that will get them to their late eighties in excellent health' but that a person
needs 'genetic booster rockets' to get to 100.

Biased attitudes towards older people

*Although my short-term memory has declined a bit I often find that
it's as good or better than many of my much younger associates.*
NEIL

The automatic linking of age and forgetfulness may play a significant role
in shaping the stereotype of ageing. Expectations of both older and younger

people can influence our thinking even when those beliefs or perceptions are unjustified. The problem with a stereotype is that it limits people to behaving in a certain way, and that in turn becomes a self-fulfilling prophecy.

The prejudice that decline was inevitable as we age was shown in a study involving two short videotapes about a character being interviewed and forgetting what the 'interviewer' had said. The two films were identical, except that in one, the 'forgetful' actor looked about 35, and in the second she looked about 75. Two separate audiences, each with a wide range of ages, then saw one of the films and afterwards wrote a short comment on the forgetful character. Overall, the mixed-age audience (who were the subjects in the study) were more likely to describe the 75-year-old character as forgetful, even though her script was exactly the same as that of the 35-year-old actor. Surprisingly perhaps, this bias was shared by older as well as younger people in the audience. In fact, the older people were even more negative about ageing. This is a telling commentary on what we are culturally encouraged to expect. It would be perfectly normal for a 75 year old to forget some things just as it is perfectly normal for younger people to forget some things.[31]

Perceptions of how old is 'old' vary with occupations. For example, female gymnasts are 'too old' in their twenties, whereas orchestral conductors are not too old in their nineties. What matters is what they can do, not what their face suggests about their age.

> *There is a wicked inclination in most people to suppose an old man decayed in his intellects. If a young or middle-aged man, when leaving a company, does not recollect where he laid his hat, it is nothing; but if the same inattention is discovered in an old man, people will shrug up their shoulders, and say, 'His memory is going'.*
> SAMUEL JOHNSON (WRITING IN 1783)[32]

Studies and tests

Existing side by side with biased expectations are the slight, but real, memory losses of ageing. In order to document which aspects of memory older people have more trouble with, tests needed to be done. However, some researchers are now finding that bias against older people has existed in traditional methods of doing studies, including leaving them out of studies altogether. This omission was partly due to a protective attitude (in case the study itself should cause the older people stress) but it meant that norms were established on younger people.

To assess the effects of ageing, two main options for studies are:

1 Will the study compare a young group of people with an older group (cross-sectional study)? or,

2 Will the study compare the same person with themselves at succeeding ages (longitudinal study)?

In a cross-sectional study (when comparing young and old) the two groups should differ only in age. They should be similar in all other aspects of their lives, such as level of education, socio-economic status, place of living, male or female and whatever other matters might influence the result of memory testing. The conditions and materials should be as comfortable and familiar to one group as to the other. Achieving this degree of impartiality is quite difficult to do.

Comparing the mental abilities of younger and older adults is much more statistically reliable if the same person is tested at successive stages in their life (the longitudinal study). Testing is ongoing at set intervals, sometimes for very many years. Any differences found between young and old would then more likely be associated with the ageing process within the individual.

Comparing one generation with another (a cross-sectional study) is confused by interference from social events, such as the type of schooling given to succeeding generations, financial depressions or boom times, or from world events like wars, or even welcome increases in medical knowledge and nutrition. The cross-sectional study is, however, valuable in some respects. Results are available quickly, rather than needing to wait for a longitudinal study to finish. Another benefit is that certain correlations, such as the relationship between intelligence and health, or educational attainment and dementia, can be noted for each age group and then compared within age groups.[33]

In order for a study to be valid, that is, to really test what it set out to test, the conditions must be controlled. A common format is to show or tell the group a list of unrelated words and then at some later time, ask for recall of the words (a task we normally don't need to do in everyday life). In order to test older and younger groups under the same conditions, participants are usually asked to go to a laboratory. This in itself can be intimidating, which in turn affects memory. In one longitudinal study, a way around the problem was found: volunteers aged between 23 and 93 years who were participating in a routine three-day period of testing (as part of the

Baltimore Longitudinal Study of Aging at the Gerontology Research Centre) were asked questions about their experiences, firstly during the study itself, then again 7 to 10 days later and again 18 to 21 months later.[34] The questions involved such things as recognising if certain materials had been on the table during the testing time, remembering how to get from the testing room to the cafeteria, and prospective/intentional memory. Older people did much better when memory tests were of this more relevant material and with no time limits. When it was important to them and they used multiple encoding, there was no difference between the older and younger people in remembering to do something in the future. Also, the whereabouts of the cafeteria and the tissues and pencils used for testing had relevance for them, whereas random strings of words did not.

When the focus of what older people try to remember is narrowed to the things that are important to them, they can compensate for age-related deficits in their memories.

Studies on how people change through adulthood

Since memory is so important in our lives, it is not surprising that its study outranks every other subject as core research in the psychology of ageing. For instance, a survey conducted from 1960 to 1980 showed articles on this topic comprised well over half of the American psychological entries in journals specialising in older people (gerontological journals).[35]

An early series of longitudinal studies began in Seattle, USA, in 1956.[36] It was an important landmark in the previously neglected study of how people change as they grow older. One of the studies found that cognitive abilities did not change much before age 60, except verbal fluency, and no differences were found between men and women.

The more ambitious Baltimore Longitudinal Study was begun in 1959, sponsored by the USA National Institute on Aging and carried out by a multidisciplinary team of researchers. The aim was to understand how people change through adulthood by testing medical, physical, learning and memory, personality and coping abilities of each individual. Large numbers of people aged from 20 to 90 years, living in the community (rather than in nursing homes or institutions), were recruited and these volunteers undertook to return every one or two years to spend several days at the Gerontology Research Clinic in Baltimore, ideally keeping to this pattern for the rest of their lives. In return they received free medical testing, which gave them knowledge of what was going on in their own bodies, and the interest of being part of ground-breaking and important studies resulting in findings that have contributed to enhancing quality of life.[37] The studies are a valuable resource in understanding what is happening in the lives of people throughout adulthood, not only in memory but in medical matters as well.

One study on memory found that there was more decline in people with less than eight years of formal education, but more than nine years of education did not necessarily confer more memory benefits. 'This suggests that a minimal amount of education during early critical periods might confer protection against cognitive decline later in life.'[38] Memory researchers continue to investigate the suggestion that early education confers benefits in later life. One plausible explanation is that more early education means a more richly connected network of brain cells, so that the slight losses of ageing are less noticeable.

The issue of why some people's memories survive better than others is still far from resolved. One Memory Survey respondent asked if the lack of use of the brain triggers memory loss. It would seem so. A finding from the Baltimore Longitudinal Study includes disuse as a possible underlying cause of memory decline. Certainly, on the positive side, continued use seems to preserve it.

Noticing memory changes on retirement

> *I wonder whether the memory loss is closely allied to the lack of urgency one experiences when you retire from your commercial vocation. [At work] you are motivated to perform at top gear. On retirement there is a strong feeling [of] 'Now I have more time'. With this feeling runs the risk if you fritter an hour here an hour there, 'so what'. So what if your mind slips down a notch and your achievement level with it. I think this is how I operate these days, I wonder if others see it my way.*
> GRANT

People often first notice a change in their memories when they reach their sixties, even though in fact recall has slowly been declining for a while. Ageing is a continuous process of change. It is not something that starts on a specific date, like retiring from a job. When people are at work and forget things, they often tell themselves they are forgetful because they are really busy. When they retire and are not busy in the same way, they expect memory to improve, but objective tests on pre- and post-retirees have shown that their memories are really just the same. At work the level of memory performance is often masked because of diaries and set routines and colleagues to jog memories. Once retired there is not the same kind of pressure to use diaries and 'to do' lists, so memory lapses are more noticeable.

Studies on retirement found that the work ethic may not be easily discarded. Some retirees could not easily relax and so evolved the 'busy ethic'. Retirement then had the same 'normal' feel as employment.[39] People who have been working set hours for perhaps 40 years have not for decades had the freedom of lengthy periods of uncommitted time, and it takes a while to find a satisfactory balance.

There are beneficial effects if a person feels in control of what happens to them. For example, one study found that if the decision to move house was out of the control of the person and the change was to a less desirable residence, then more illness was associated with retirement.[40]

Retiring doesn't change the brain, but it does change how one uses it, and the structure of the day. Retiring from work doesn't mean retiring from life. One just changes gears, and hats.

Twenty-first century retirees relish their better health and freedom to do things. It comes, therefore, as something of a shock to notice changes in memory and speaking fluency, particularly as one feels perfectly competent in other ways.[41] Confidence can be restored with understanding that a certain amount of decline of some aspects of the memory system is normal for older people. It is not a sure sign of worse to come and certainly not a reason to withdraw from previous activities or refrain from learning new ones.

Memory abilities of older and younger people

… youth goes right on growing old.[42]

Overall, some differences are noticeable in the memory abilities of younger and older people but there are also large differences in attitudes to memory lapses. Younger people are much more likely to skip lightly over forgetfulness whereas older people worry about its significance. However, age can bring increased emotional stability with more positive feelings and fewer negative ones. Older people can use this asset to organise their lives and use their memories more wisely.

Variability in ageing patterns

Variability is the hallmark of normal ageing.[43]

Patterns in ageing clearly distinguish common ageing processes from illnesses. Mild decline in memory and other abilities is part of the normal ageing process. Within this norm there are some interesting patterns and variations. Everybody does not age in exactly the same way.

Since memory cannot be fully understood in isolation from the rest of the body, the three patterns of ageing outlined below include physiological as well as mental patterns:[44]

1   One pattern is the stereotype of a regular, linear decline in some physiological functions while others remain quite stable until very late in the life span.

2   Another common pattern is that physiological loss only occurs when a person develops an age-related illness such as heart disease. If there is no heart disease, the heart pumps as well at 70 as it did at 30 years of age (and a good memory is dependent upon a good blood supply to the brain).

3   The next pattern is that loss of brain cells does occur but is compensated for by built-in mechanisms. Connections between brain cells (neurons) can grow longer and develop more branches, presumably as a result of continuing mental activity by the person.

Not everyone fits neatly into one of these three patterns and people may show a combination of more than one.

The senses[45]

Everything we know and remember about the world outside our bodies comes to us via the senses. What we hear, see, smell, taste and feel is initially the only means we have of knowing what's out there in the world and how it may affect us.

All our learning via the senses is in constant conversation with our planning, considering and evaluating brain areas. Therefore memory and indeed all aspects of life are vitally affected by the conditions of the senses. All senses diminish with age but the extent of the losses varies between senses and between individuals.

Hearing

I blame deteriorating hearing for forgetting what I am told,
particularly when there is a lot of incidental other noise and speech.
ARTHUR

An intact hearing system provides the ability to tune in and out to particular sounds, such as tuning in to what one person is saying when there is other noise around. When hearing deteriorates we do miss the ability to exclude unwanted background noise. In general, hearing deteriorates from age 55, with high-pitched sounds being lost first. A survey in the UK found that 92 per cent of people over 60 years had at least some significant hearing loss.[46] The cause can be due to deterioration of the various structures of the inner ear, or with the auditory areas of the brain. A common cause of deafness is a build-up of wax in the outer ear, easily removed by a doctor syringing with a steady stream of warm water.

Poor hearing has a very isolating effect on a person, but compensatory measures can be taken. Some kinds of deafness are helped by using a hearing aid. There is a range of modern digital hearing aids suited to various needs by means of a tiny computer chip. They fit unobtrusively in or behind the ear and can be regulated on the spot according to the amount of background noise or to more clearly hear the person directly in front of the wearer. Digital hearing aids are also compatible with high-quality digital telephones.

Sight

An enormous amount of brain space is given to processing the endless succession of images that we see. Our visual memories then become our own reconstructions, so no two people will have exactly the same visual memories, even after looking at the same scene.

Vision relies on the incoming image being detected as variations in light and colour by the light-sensitive membrane at the back of the eye, the retina. As we age there are gradual changes in the eye: the retina needs more light to see the image; the cornea, the tough transparent covering to the eye, becomes less transparent and begins to flatten; the lens behind the pupil can become more opaque (called a cataract); and there is less flexibility in the tiny muscles that control the iris and hence the size of the pupil.

Few people have perfect sight and many deficiencies can be corrected by prescription spectacles. However, with ageing, a major concern is to optimise the vision we do have, treating conditions such as cataracts and detecting preventable diseases, such as glaucoma, early. Glaucoma is due to a build up of pressure that slowly destroys the optic nerve at the back of the eye and is insidious because we are not aware of it.[47] A change in eyesight can be expected about every five years but even people with good eyesight should still have routine checks every two years for early detection of preventable problems.

Vision is tightly integrated with the rest of the brain. The retina has a small central area known as the macula and its degeneration can affect reading and focussing directly in front of the eyes. A little known phenomenon is that visual hallucinations (called the Charles Bonnet syndrome) can result from macular degeneration.[48] People can 'see' bizarre things like monkeys sitting on people's laps or fire engines in a hospital ward. The person knows they are not real but may not know they are caused by failing eyesight, rather than a breakdown in rational function.

TASTE AND SMELL

There are only four types of tastebuds – sweet, salty, sour and bitter – but they can detect minute amounts of a substance. Different combinations give appetising variation to our cooking. We have excellent memories for unpleasant tastes. Any attempt to lessen the taste of a bitter medicine – for example, by adding orange juice – is liable to register a dislike of orange juice. The sense of taste deteriorates by about age 40 to 50. The flavour of food can be enhanced by adding herbs and spices and through our sense of smell.

Smells have a powerful ability to remind us of some long-past experience. The pleasant, pungent odour of wet bushland reminds one couple we know of good walks they have had together and they say to each other: 'They're playing our smell again.'

A surprisingly large area of the brain is devoted to processing smells, given our perception that it is not one of our most important senses. Articles on how to sell your home suggest brewing coffee and baking bread in the kitchen and putting lavender sachets in the cupboards. Traces of these scents bring a homey feeling of well-being to prospective buyers that is outside their conscious awareness, so they might well feel an emotional preference to your house over others.

The ability to distinguish very many different smells remains intact until about age 65, even if the different smells can't be identified. The loss of sense of smell in older age is very gradual and may not be noticed very much by the person. As with taste, there does not seem to be any remedial action that can be taken.

Touch and equilibrium

Touch and our internal sense of equilibrium (position and balance) are the senses that tell us about the relationship of our body to the outside world. Nerve impulses from the soles of the feet plus information from joints (giving position sense) plus information from the inner ear and vision combine to tell us which way is up, and connections to the muscular system keep us upright. Equilibrium is less efficient in ageing, and older people have a higher risk of falling when their reflexes become slower. Exercise can improve a sense of balance.

How people shape their lives

> *Just as our thinking affects how we act, the reverse may be equally true. How we actually behave can produce marked cognitive change.*[49]

The pattern of creativity appears to be relatively independent of physical patterns. Anyone can have creative potential and even in later years can generate new combinations of ideas in artistic endeavour.[50] Geniuses begin their creative work early in life and continue till late in life, often in spite of massive problems. Beethoven and Bedrich Smetana continued composing in spite of not being able to hear their own music, and the blind mathematician Leonhard Euler did his complex calculations totally in his head.

Side by side with the physical happenings of our lives is the ability we have to mould, even in some small way, our lives to suit us. One of the Baltimore studies set out to investigate how the world shaped people from the age of 20 years as they grew older but instead they discovered that the reverse was happening: people could shape their world to fit them.[51] People's everyday decisions and actions influence the directions their lives take and the cumulative effect over the years strengthens their identity.

New brain cell connections

> *I am particularly concerned as to whether our brain cells die off as we age.*
> **HARRIETT**

As we age we do lose brain cells but not necessarily in significant numbers and not across the board.[52] We are born with a staggeringly large number so we can afford to lose a few.

Every part of our bodies is made up of cells which have a limited life span and then die. Although brain cells do not normally reproduce themselves, an exciting discovery from the last decade is that they can grow new branches, which are the connections to other cells.[53] Such growth of new connections – dendrites – is thought to compensate for the loss of neighbouring cells.[54]

The latest research also suggests that adult brains may even retain some special cells that, under the right conditions, can develop into new brain cells. (For more details see Chapter 8, 'The Brain in Action').

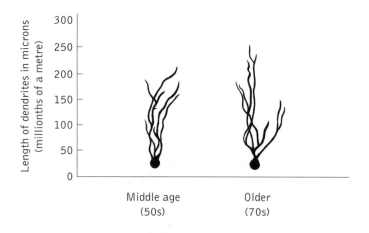

Older people can grow new branches to their brain cells.[55]

Chronological age or biological age

Mac (a friend) was enthusing about exceptional 90 year olds he has known, among them his mother and a retired university professor. The common denominator, reflected Mac, was their attitude, the expectation that life was interesting and they meant to take part in it.

The older we get, the less that chronological age (the number of years since we were born) will indicate how well we are functioning. Biological age is the measure of how we actually feel and act. Anecdotal evidence suggests that people of 90 years and over who garden, play music, mountain climb or do something out of the ordinary for their age, function at a much younger chronological age. One of the key attributes seems to be their positive attitudes and flexible approach to life.

At a glance

- In normal ageing, aspects of memory that stay good are knowledge-based (semantic), priming and existing physical skills.

- Aspects of memory that worsen with age are forming new memories of specific events (episodic) and learning new physical skills.

- Memory is improved by allowing extra time, by avoiding competing demands for attention and by the provision of recognition cues to recall.

- The memory that underpins our enduring sense of self is maintained well with age.

- Vivid memories from long ago are reconstructions so the gist is likely to be more accurate than the details.

- Memory is a major area of gerontology research. Longitudinal and cross-sectional studies are investigating the range of variability in ageing patterns.

- Senses like sight and hearing are important channels for bringing outside information into the mind. Losses are gradual and often hardly noticed but regular checkups, particularly of eyesight, can detect and help remedy problems early.

- Brain cells can grow new connections throughout life and new brain cells may even develop in special regions when we mentally exercise.

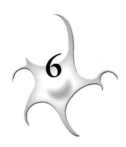

Normal Memory Loss or Alzheimer's?

Normal memory loss and amnesia due to Alzheimer's disease involve different kinds of changes in the brain. This means that the next time you forget where you put your car keys, you need not worry that you are headed towards Alzheimer's. Nor do you need to become concerned the next time you fail to come up with the name of a friend that feels like it is on the tip of your tongue. But if you forget that you possess a car or you can't remember your own name, then there is clearly cause for concern.[1]

Many of our Memory Survey respondents feared that benign memory loss might lead into dementia. One respondent asked: 'Is there a continuum between slight memory loss and incapacitated memory loss?' The answer is no. Memory loss in normal ageing might get worse from about the age of 60, but it doesn't include the diseases known as dementia.

The term 'dementia' is a blanket term covering any loss of mental ability that can impair a person's ability to function, and does not include the small losses of brain cells due to normal ageing. The most common type of dementia in older adults is Alzheimer's disease, which progressively damages the nerve cells of the brain and causes the slow loss of memory among other cognitive abilities.[2]

When a person has memory loss, two main points to consider are:

1 Minor memory losses do not impair a person's ability to look after themselves. In normal ageing, memory problems fluctuate, often due to a variety of reasons such as tiredness, stress, or poor health. With remedy to these causes, memory improves.

2 In Alzheimer's disease, memory problems may fluctuate from day to day but typically get gradually worse over time, becoming noticeable to an objective observer over a period of some months.

Difficulties with diagnosing Alzheimer's

The diagnosis of Alzheimer's disease is difficult, because in the very early stages many other curable conditions can look the same. These include vitamin deficiency, infection, thyroid deficiency, stress and depression. More serious, but often treatable, are heart conditions, stroke, and tumours.[3]

Currently a diagnosis can only indicate that the dementia is probably Alzheimer's and hence the term 'dementia of the Alzheimer's type' (DAT) is used. In general, episodic memory is badly affected, but eventually all areas are affected.[4] The diagnosis of DAT is not given unless several other areas of brain function as well as memory are affected and decline is progressive over several months. Until recently it could only be confirmed by a post-mortem although this may change in the near future.

When post-mortems have been done, people who had DAT typically have many plaques and tangles in their brains. Senile plaques are patches of diseased tissue that contain clumps of abnormal proteins surrounded by the debris of degenerating brain cells. There are different kinds of plaques, such as amyloid plaques, named after the hard lumps of amyloid (a type of protein) at their centre. Neurofibrillary tangles are abnormally twisted filaments inside brain cells. Plaques and tangles are found in the brains of normally ageing people to a small degree but not in the same high concentrations as in DAT.

In the early stages of DAT there are high concentrations of plaques and tangles in the regions most closely associated with episodic memory, in particular, the input to the hippocampus. By contrast, a different area involved in processing the output of the hippocampus is associated with the minor memory losses in ordinary ageing, and the majority of people with age-related memory loss do not develop dementia.[5]

> *One of my biggest fears is to suffer from dementia later on. (My mother suffered dementia in her later years – she lived to be 80.)*
> IRIS

A large number of the Memory Survey respondents said that they could cope with their current forgetfulness, but dreaded that it was leading to Alzheimer's disease. Our purpose in this chapter is to describe the known differences for the relief of people who only have benign forgetting, and to suggest ways of seeking help for those who think they may be in the very early stages of dementia disease. Scraps of misinformation about dementia are circulated by word of mouth. Such misinformation is damaging because it is denigrating, needlessly scary, or perpetuates wrong information. As the Alzheimer's Association explains, 'Older age presents a risk factor, but is not the cause of dementia ... Loss of memory in dementia is more than just becoming a little forgetful. It is persistent and progressive, not just occasional.'[6]

Myths about memory

There are plenty of half-truths about memory which are circulated by word of mouth. We call them myths. They have some small substance but are old beliefs that have not yet caught up with scientific discoveries of the last decade or so. Here are some common myths or half-truths:

- 'Everyone gets Alzheimer's when old.' Wrong. The vast majority of people don't. This misconception is not helped by the jocular saying 'I must be getting Alzheimer's' every time a person forgets some trifling thing.

- 'If one of your parents had Alzheimer's, you will get it too.' Not so. The early onset form of the disease (before age 65) is thought to be hereditary but even then the environment plays a part in whether the disease develops.[7]

- 'If you could only do one thing to boost your brain power, do crosswords.' Useful advice (but not the best). If there is only time for one thing on any given day, walk or do aerobic exercises for at least 20 minutes to get that blood supply coursing through the brain. Brain cells need oxygen.[8]

- 'You don't have to do anything about it in the very early stages of Alzheimer's disease.' This is head-in-the-sand thinking. Medical assessment is needed to assess if it really is dementia, and if it is, get prescription medications as early as possible to delay its progression.

- 'There would be no hope for me if I was diagnosed with probable A.D.' Unfair to yourself. Early diagnosis is important so that appropriate medications can be taken to slow the rate of the disease and help memory and everyday living.

The trouble with half-truths is that there is just enough fact in them to grab the attention, but not enough truth to give an accurate picture of what is happening or what should be done.

Percentage of population at risk

For someone under the age of 65, the chance of getting a dementia disease in the next year is much less than one in a hundred. The incidence rises to about 6 to 8 per hundred for people over the age of 85. There are frequent references in the media to 1 in 5 (or 20 per cent), but this percentage refers to a 25-year period. In any one year, everyone over 65 has (on average) a very high chance of not *getting it.*[9]

Alzheimer's and other dementia diseases are a major health problem for communities in Australia and worldwide. However, some people have over-estimated their chances of contracting the disease because in many reports a distinction is not made between the total number of people with Alzheimer's in a population and the average number of people likely to contract the disease in any one year. The population is ageing, which does mean that there are more people getting dementia but there are also more people ageing healthily (largely due to a reduction in heart disease).[10]

In medical terms, the number of people who already have Alzheimer's is the 'prevalence' of the disease. The number of new cases in any one year is the 'incidence' of the disease. If a government health department wanted to know the number of nursing home places needed by Alzheimer's patients, they would need to know the prevalence – how many patients already had the disease.[11] But if an individual is concerned about their own health, they will be much more interested in the incidence – the number of probable new cases in the next year. As noted above, the incidence is very low for people under 65. The risks increase up to the age of 90, but some studies show that they may decline after that, and dementia is common but not inevitable for 100 year olds.[12] As the UK Alzheimer's Society explains, 'Dementia is not an inevitable consequence of old age. Most 90 year olds, for example, do not have the condition.'[13]

It seems clear that lifestyle plays some role in the development of dementia diseases. Consistent with this idea, the relative rates of different types of dementias vary between countries. In Australia, Europe and the USA, Alzheimer's is the most common type, whereas in Asian countries it is less common. In Japan vascular dementia is twice as frequent as Alzheimer's, but follows the Western pattern in the children of people who moved from Japan to Hawaii. In Australia, dementia is the third highest cause of disability among women (after heart disease and stroke) and the fifth highest cause among men (after heart disease, stroke, lung cancer and respiratory diseases).[14] Factors that are associated with increased prevalence of Alzheimer's, apart from age, include level of education, previous head injuries, diet and lifestyle, and some genetic factors (see the section later in this chapter 'About genes' for details).[15]

Comparing normal changes with Alzheimer's

In the ageing process, people often notice slight deterioration in their own memories and sometimes other body states, which can be confused with the very early stages of Alzheimer's. To understand these changes, it helps to divide everyday functioning into four broad areas:

1   Intellectual processing – thinking and reasoning.

2   Language – talking and listening.

3   Feeling – social and emotional abilities.

4   Physical – movement and body control.

For each of these areas, contrasting the normal ageing response with a typical response a person with DAT makes the differences much clearer.

1 Thinking and reasoning

[I forget] where I put things, especially now that I have recently moved from a 2 bed, big kitchen to a small 1 bed.
RUTH

Normal: For normally ageing people, a new situation like moving can cause a dramatic alteration in their routine, so that they need extra time to remember where all their things are now kept. They can learn. It's not always easy, but the challenge can be met. Brain cells can make new connections, even in older brains. Being temporarily overwhelmed can cause dementia-like symptoms and the person may need professional help in overcoming it. Other causes of temporary dementia-like symptoms may be a too heavy workload, stress, medication or depression, which are all treatable.

A person with DAT: People with DAT don't seem to be able to profit by the strategy of deliberate attention to making associations.[16] For example, a couple bought a new stove, which had the on/off knobs in a different position from the old stove. The wife said, 'I can't work that', and she could not learn the new relationship of switches to elements and did no more cooking from then on. Relatives said that giving up in this way was so unlike her.

ORGANISING

Normal: Tidying up a disorganised cupboard or garage is a job we tend to put off, but when we do get around to it, we can get the job done methodically. A big job may need some planning on paper, perhaps with lists or a concept map.

A person with DAT: An elderly lady living with her equally elderly husband went to the bathroom each night to shower. She changed her clothes regularly. The trouble was the dirty clothes went straight back into the drawers, missing out the laundry circuit completely. The still alert husband did not notice, even though he did the washing.

Although there is variation between different people in the exact location of initial brain deterioration in Alzheimer's, it is sometimes worst in the front part of the brain, which deals with what is called executive behaviour: planning, organising, and sorting.

Normal: Checking the change when shopping is a fairly routine matter for most of us and is not too difficult. A person might not check their change every time, particularly when rushed, but could if they wanted to.

A person with DAT: When shopping a woman with DAT was regularly putting the change away in her purse without looking at it. When urged to check it, she said that she could not count it. When making sandwiches for three people, the same woman became confused and distressed when she couldn't count out two slices of bread per person. Someone with dementia could 'forget completely what the numbers are and what needs to be done with them'.[17]

2 Talking and listening

REMEMBERING WORDS

Normal: Everyone has trouble finding the right word sometimes; for example, one survey respondent wrote, 'Words are elusive … I try to concentrate solely on the lost memory, knowing I do know the answer – it just has to be found.' If a person doesn't remember a name when they want to, but does remember it later, it shows that the problem is mainly with cues for recall and the information is not lost.

A person with DAT: A person with DAT may forget simple words or substitute inappropriate words, making sentences incomprehensible, or may fail to encode names or make sense of the sounds of language. Christine Boden writes of 'problems understanding what people say on the phone and who they are, and remembering the names for things and people.'[18]

3 Social and emotional abilities

DEALING WITH OTHER PEOPLE

Normal: Our social lives include behaving appropriately in social situations and recognising our friends and maintaining our friendships. We share in their joys and feel anxiety on their behalf if they are in trouble.

A person with DAT: A person with DAT can feel worried in social situations without knowing why, and without understanding those feelings. They may withdraw from social life and lose contact with former friends.

Expressing and dealing with emotions

Normal: Our emotional lives include feeling a range of emotions, but we can control the public expression of feelings of frustration and anger. Most people feel thoroughly irritated and frustrated and perhaps suspicious at times but can recognise those feelings in themselves and deal with both the feelings and the situation in a socially acceptable way. We can also share our feelings with loved ones.

A person with DAT: A person with DAT may show inappropriate emotion; for example, laughing at the sad point in a film or having periods of uncontrollable crying which they cannot explain. They may show rapid mood swings from impatience and restlessness to dull and apathetic; or they may react aggressively and suspiciously, even, as the disease progresses, to those who love them and care for them. Feelings of distress, particularly about memory loss, may be denied.

4 Movement and body control

Remembering how to do things

Normal: In normal ageing, people don't forget how to do the things they do often, like drive a car or use tools or household appliances, or how to post a letter. Procedural memory takes care of the learning and retention of the things we know how to do.

People with poor eyesight might sometimes let crockery fall through misjudging how far away a shelf is, or if they have arthritis in their hands they might have difficulty doing up buttons, but they understand what the difficulties are and generally remain in control of body movements.

A person with DAT: As one friend told us, 'My mother used to be able to do sewing with tiny stitches. One day when helping her dress, I found her singlet mended with great cobbled stitches so that it would not go over her head. She had no idea what the problem was.' In another situation, with all the neighbours on board, ready to drive to church, a woman sat in the driver's seat of a car with the ignition key in her hand and said that she had forgotten how to start the car.

People with DAT might have difficulty doing up buttons and putting on clothes in the right order. They may forget how to carry out the movements needed to get dressed, or how to take care of their clothes. Surprisingly, however, even in an advanced stage of the disease, some abilities may be spared, such as how to sing, or the physical movements needed for golf. The pattern of what is lost can differ markedly between different people.

Normal: It is normal for someone to forget for a few moments where they are, for example when driving, but they can quickly flip back into recognition of a familiar landscape; or if they are out walking, they don't forget what their own street looks like.

A person with DAT: People with DAT can become lost while driving on a familiar route, not knowing where they are or how to get home again, or they may find their own street quite unfamiliar.

Coping with everyday activities

In normal ageing, everyday memory problems can be frustrating, but they don't pose a threat to a person's ability to do things for themselves and to live independently in their own home. One ongoing study asked participants to assess their own ability to take care of themselves and their responses were then compared to objective assessments. The conclusion was that the participants' own assessments were accurate.[19]

> *The events and changes in the life of a person with early stage dementia who has yet to be diagnosed are generally only recognised as significant in retrospect. Something might happen that is slotted into the basket called 'Yes, but we all do that sometimes' and is promptly forgotten. It is only when a second or third incident occurs, or maybe someone at work or home makes a comment about a behaviour, mood or loss of a skill, that medical help is sought.*[20]

When carers of people with DAT search their memories for the earliest signs that their loved one was not remembering well, they will typically give an example with the comment: 'It was so unlike him or her'. As the months or years pass, a person with DAT will gradually require increasing assistance with everyday activities that they used to do by themselves, such as taking a bath or writing a cheque. There may be a danger of inappropriate behaviour, such as trying to heat water in a plastic basin on a gas flame. They might put on several shirts or blouses, put things in grossly inappropriate places such as reading glasses with the sugar in the sugar bowl, or sprinkle cold ashes over the carpet as though it was the garden.

The vast majority of people don't develop dementia, but nearly everybody does develop some memory lapses as part of the normal ageing process. Knowledge about a normally functioning brain is important to our understanding of what is beyond the range of normal. However, note that the comparisons in this section are intended to inform in a general way. They cannot substitute for individual assessment from a professional.[21]

Where to go for help

I even went to my GP some years ago, very afraid that I was in the early stages of Alzheimer's disease, my memory was such a problem – he laughed at me. I do have a lot on my plate so I realise at this age specially a lot of things must 'fall off'.

ANTONIA

There are many sources of help for people with continuing memory concerns. In recent years medical research has made enormous progress in developing diagnostic tools that give accurate information about the condition of the brain and medications to help people with dementia. If the diagnosis is something else, again there may be remedies for what really is the matter. The process of clarification begins with a visit to a general practitioner (GP), who will refer the person to specialists if necessary.

The person or a concerned relative may want to ask a GP for a referral to a neuropsychologist – a psychologist who specialises in things that go wrong with the brain.

Diagnosis may involve several things, including a simple test of everyday knowledge, designed to cover all aspects of memory and thinking. Examples are the Mini-Mental State Test and the Silly Sentences test, which can be given by a general practitioner, a geriatrician, or a brain specialist such as a neurologist or neuropsychologist. Newer tests, such as the Herman Buschke test, show promise for discriminating between Alzheimer's disease and age-related memory loss in the early stages, but have yet to be used widely in general practice.[22]

Specialists

A **neuropsychologist** is a psychologist who specialises in things that go wrong with the brain, and provides advice on how to cope with life made difficult by a neurological disease such as dementia.

A **neurologist** or **neurophysician** is a medical doctor who specialises in brain problems such as migraines or epilepsy, and may prescribe medications.

A **neuropsychiatrist** is a medical doctor who specialises in the kinds of brain abnormalities that cause serious disruption to independent living.

A **neuroscientist** is a scientist, engineer or medical specialist who is involved in any area of brain research.

A **geriatrician** is a medical doctor who specialises in caring for older people.

A **general practitioner** is a specialist in knowing which type of specialist to refer a patient to!

The Mini-Mental State Test[23]

The Mini-Mental State Test is a standardised test widely used by the medical profession in an initial assessment of a person 'at risk'. Here are some of the questions:

> What is the date?   Where are we?
>
> Count backwards by 7s, beginning at 100, for at least 5 subtractions OR spell WORLD backwards.

The person will be shown items in everyday use such as a wristwatch or pencil and asked to name them. They will also be asked to copy this design:

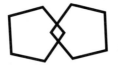
In the scoring, wobbly lines don't matter but the figures must intersect and each have five sides.

The full test includes more questions of the same sort, and is not difficult for someone whose brain is not damaged by disease. In fact we think the hardest question is knowing the date! The questions test all areas of cognitive function, not just memory. There is no ethical problem with us telling you about the test because anyone with established dementia of the Alzheimer's type would find the test very difficult and would not be helped by seeing the questions in advance. Even in normal ageing there is variation between individual performance over the years on the Mini-Mental State Test. For some people, it seems normal to score about one point less per decade. For others (still in the normal range), there is little loss before the age of 60, then a slightly bigger loss after that.[24]

SILLY SENTENCES TEST

The following sentences are examples of those used in the Silly Sentences test, which tests semantic memory.[25] In this test, the person is asked to decide if the sentence is a sensible or a silly one.

Pork chops can be bought in shops	yes or no?
Jamaica is edible	yes or no?
Oranges drill teeth	yes or no?

People with damage to brain areas which store semantic memory find the Silly Sentences test difficult because those areas store general knowledge and understanding of what objects are used for.

Brain imaging techniques

> It is not an exaggeration to say that the new technologies of neuroimaging have revolutionised this approach to the study of memory, and that the area is one of the most exciting and dynamic in present-day science.[26]

The techniques of brain imaging (or neuroimaging) can help to pinpoint particular areas of the brain. Comparisons can be made between regions in normally functioning brains and those showing problems. Before brain imaging techniques were developed and used effectively, knowledge about brain areas was slowly built up with records of people who had accidents or damage to some part of their brains. The knowledge was used to help patients as much as possible. Eventually the records could be matched up with information from post-mortem examinations.

Diagnosis of brain problems can now be helped by the use of modern, non-intrusive methods of brain imaging – the 'revolution' referred to in the above quotation.

CAT SCANS

CAT (computerised axial tomography) scans were the earliest type of brain scan, first used in the early 1970s.[28] They use X-rays to scan the brain and other tissues, taking a series of 'photographs' at very precise distances from the 'camera'. It's a bit like thinly slicing a block of ice cream that has swirls of chocolate and strawberry through it. At each slice, a different pattern is revealed. The two-dimensional slices are then converted by a computer program to a three-dimensional image.

PET SCANS AND fMRI

PET (positron emission tomography) scanning and fMRI (functional magnetic resonance imaging) are more technologically sophisticated than a CAT scan. Both methods work by measuring blood flow to a particular area of the brain as those cells become active.[29] Brain cells must have nourishment in the form of oxygen and glucose carried to them by the bloodstream. When a certain group of the brain's nerve cells work hard – that is, all fire as the person is thinking – the extra blood flow to that area can be measured. Those measurements are transferred to a computer screen, and coloured to indicate areas of stronger or weaker activity. In the most common form of PET scan, a radioactive marker is injected into the bloodstream. For safety reasons there is a limit to the number of times this can be done to any one person in a single year.

Recently, PET scans have been used to make images of the plaques and tangles typically found in the brains of people with advanced DAT. Previously, the presence of plaques and tangles could only be established at autopsy, but a way has been found to inject a living person with a radioactive tracer that binds to plaques and tangles. The PET scan can then find and image them. It is hoped that the technique will lead to early diagnosis of Alzheimer's disease, enabling doctors to fine-tune and monitor treatments more exactly.[30]

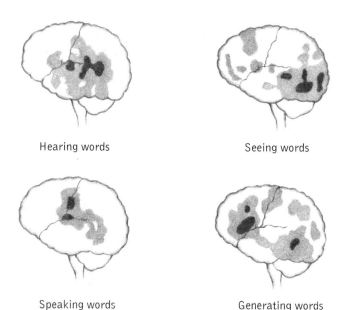

Hearing words

Seeing words

Speaking words

Generating words

PET scans showing brain maps of areas that became more active when a normally functioning person heard, saw, spoke and thought up words to say. The increased activity is shown by the dark areas.[31]

fMRI is a later invention and gives the clearest picture of the tissues. The patient lies in a tunnel with a strong magnetic field all around. The machine makes radio waves – heard as loud beeps – which cause measurable changes in the atoms of the tissues as they respond to the magnetism.[32] As in PET scans, fMRI measures blood flow to the area where the brain cells are functioning as the patient concentrates upon whatever the examiner requests, for example: 'Imagine lifting your hand to use a hammer.' The latest scanners can produce images speedily (four every second), which aids in understanding which areas of the brain are more active during each mental task.

MEG SCANS

MEG (magnetoencephalography) scans work by measuring the tiny electrical signals emitted by brain cells as they fire and alert nearby cells. MEG works more accurately and more quickly than its predecessors for the outside cortical brain layers. Its limitations are that it is not so effective for the deeper layer of brain signals.[33]

Is aluminium still implicated in Alzheimer's?

A link between aluminium and Alzheimer's disease was first suggested when it was found in the brains of people affected. It is now thought to be a secondary association rather than a cause – that is, something that can occur with Alzheimer's disease but does not cause it. Comparisons have been made with people who have kidney failure and cannot excrete aluminium. Even after years of treatments that contain aluminium, those people did not develop Alzheimer's.

Researchers believe that, in the majority of those affected, Alzheimer's disease results from a combination of different risk factors rather than a single cause. Such factors, which vary from person to person, may include age, genetic predisposition, other diseases or environmental agents.

ALZHEIMER'S SOCIETY[27]

Medications

I try so very hard for the short time I am with you that you would hardly know I was ill ... After you have gone I sink back exhausted, monosyllabic, wrung out and empty of all showmanship. It may take me a least a few hours lying down with my eyes closed to recover ... And, of course, all of this assumes I am taking my tablets, the tacrine ... When I don't take them, and it is all too easy for me to forget them, then the world goes too fast for me. I can't even pretend to be 'normal'. I'm off-line, unable to speak or to think, lost in a foggy confusion.

CHRISTINE BODEN (WHO HAD EARLY ONSET ALZHEIMER'S DISEASE)[34]

People with DAT can have shortages of the chemical messengers (neurotransmitters) which pass between the cells of the brain. One such neurotransmitter is acetylcholine, essential for the proper working of some areas concerned with memory. A variety of medications are available to help relieve the symptoms caused by the shortages. Some work by boosting a particular class of neurotransmitters – for example, tacrine slows the breakdown of acetylcholine in the junctions between cells. Other medications called vasodilators improve blood flow to the brain, either by expanding the blood vessels directly or by stimulating the brain's metabolism. Response to the medications varies from large benefits for a small number of people, to no noticeable difference for others.

It is theoretically possible to give a neurotransmitter booster in pill form. However, the body's natural protection system makes it very difficult to get these substances to where they could be of use – that is, right into the cells. Brain cells are protected by the special construction of the blood vessel walls, usually known as the 'blood-brain barrier'. Many 'foreign' substances carried by the bloodsteam can't get through, which unfortunately includes most medications. One exception is the neurotransmitter dopamine, which is used to treat Parkinson's disease. Dopamine is converted to a substance called L-DOPA, which can pass from blood vessels through the wall into brain cells where it is converted back to dopamine.[35]

New and improved treatments are continually being researched and becoming available to patients. Research also continues into areas that may preserve brain cells, including the roles of anti-inflammatory agents and antioxidants. For a readable discussion of treatment possibilities, see Howard Gruetzner's comprehensive book, *Alzheimer's: The Complete Guide for Families and Loved Ones*.[36]

Support for people with DAT and for carers

Large public hospitals have geriatric teams that provide education, counselling and support. The geriatric team is multi-disciplinary and can include the family's GP, a neuropsychologist, neurophysician, social worker, occupational therapist and speech therapist.[37] At a first request, some of the team will go to a person's home and help them assess the situation and offer help and advice. They can also organise short-term respite care, which often functions like a social club, involving outdoor activities such as picnics, a mild version of cricket, or just throwing a ball around. Indoor activities might include discussing the current news with a leader who goes through a daily newspaper, doing crosswords, playing scrabble or cooking. More energetic activities might be indoor bowls or sticky darts.

A major advantage of respite care is that the carer has some time off to have a rest, get some relaxation or just do their own thing. Meetings are also organised monthly for carers, with discussion groups and sometimes a video.

THE ALZHEIMER'S ASSOCIATION

A friend's sister has dementia and can no longer cook. Her husband is finding the going hard. When we suggested the Alzheimer's Association, our friend replied, 'Oh she's not that bad yet', which suggests to us that the role of the Alzheimer's Association may not be well understood in the community.

Support and information for people with dementia of the Alzheimer's type and carers is available from the Alzheimer's Association in each capital city. Its services include:

- use of their lending library of videos and courses

- a quarterly newsletter containing brief reviews of research and associated news

- a help line, linking people into support groups

- information about respite care, counselling, seminars and information meetings, and

- a web page (see addresses in the references at the end of this chapter).

Anyone may join the association, as we did when we began writing this book. The Alzheimer's Association has an extensive library which visitors may use, and organises seminars, such as 'Health and Safety for Family Carers', 'Nutrition throughout Dementia' and 'Activities for People with Dementia'.

The quarterly publication *InTouch* features a page called 'Research Briefs' written by Dr Helen Creasey and Professor Henry Brodaty, honorary medical advisers to the Alzheimer's Association of NSW. They comment realistically on some of the eye-catching media headlines, which often turn out to be about hopes for the future or plans for studies as yet untested. 'Research Briefs' also gives news and evaluations about the latest research into the disease and its treatment.[38]

Ongoing research

> … *research into DAT is now one of the biggest single areas of biomedical research.*[39]

At a recent international conference on Alzheimer's disease, over two thousand research papers were presented on the different approaches being taken for diagnosis, treatment, risk factors and interventions.[40] Promising new approaches include a technique for imaging amyloid plaques using PET scans and searches for more Alzheimer's susceptibility genes.

Risk factors for developing Alzheimer's currently being studied include a wide range of effects such as diet, cholesterol levels, body weight, physical exercise, mental activity and social contact. Recent epidemiological studies of diet and lifestyle indicate that certain types of diet can substantially lower the risk of developing Alzheimer's. In general, factors that contribute to heart disease also seem to be risk factors for Alzheimer's (see the next chapter for details of risk factors and how to lower them).

Current research into treatment options include supplying key missing chemicals to the brain, and even transplanting key genes. Other approaches included development of a vaccine against Alzheimer's when tests on mice showed that it was possible. Initial trials with people were discontinued when they developed inflammation of the brain but the search for a safe vaccine is still an area of active research.[41]

Genes and chromosomes

Our bodies are formed of cells. Within each cell are the genes that provide the biochemical blueprint for a person's characteristics. Genes also run the body throughout life. They are organised into groups on 23 pairs of chromosomes, each identified by a number. As a body grows, each cell multiplies by dividing into two daughter cells, each one with a full set of chromosomes. Although all cells contain the same set of genes, different types of cells express, or activate, only a small subset at any one time. In very recent times the worldwide genome project has mapped 30,000 human genes. This is a mind-blowing achievement, but does not tell us what each gene does nor what happens if it is damaged.

More about genes

Many genes are of special interest to Alzheimer's researchers. Some make precursor proteins to amyloid (the protein in the plaques that are characteristic of the disease).[42] Others appear to be agents of clean-up operations that remove toxic protein fragments from around brain cells. As is the case with most genes, different versions of these genes exist (called alleles). Some of them make slight variations of the same protein, but others are damaged so that they do not function at all. Since each person has two copies of each gene (one from each parent), they could have the same allele twice, or two different ones.

In different people, Alzheimer's may be associated with damage to different parts of the chain of events that controls the production and scavenging of the toxic amyloid protein.[43] In families with members that have the rare early-onset forms of the disease (typically aged in their forties and fifties), mutations that lead to abnormal processing of the amyloid precursor protein have been found in genes on chromosomes 1, 14 and 21. In the more common late-onset forms, the situation is more complex and some cases of Alzheimer's seem to run in families, although most cases have no known genetic component. Studying the genetic forms may help explain what is happening in the non-familial forms. One suggestion is that genes related to clean-up operations may be factors in the late-onset familial cases, including genes for the proteins ApoE (on chromosome 19) and A2M (on chromosome 12). Different forms of these genes are associated with different levels of risk.[44]

Some gene variants protect and others predispose a person to a particular disease – but it should be noted that 'predisposing' is not the same as causing a disease. For example, fair skin is more susceptible to sunburn, but whether a person gets sunburnt depends on their environment, not just their genes, and not having fair skin does not protect against sunburn. Similarly, decreased blood flow may be partially mitigated by increased exercise and good diet. A recent epidemiological study has shown that elevated cholesterol and blood pressure place a person at a greater risk of developing Alzheimer's than even the most risky variant of ApoE (E4).[45]

Much is still to be discovered about the causes of Alzheimer's, and there may be a role for environmental factors such as antioxidants and anti-inflammatory drugs that may slow the development of the disease, possibly by interrupting the cell-damaging effects of the amyloid plaques.

In summary, the genetics of Alzheimer's is complex and estimates vary widely on the relative importance of genes compared to other factors.[46] Not everyone with one or more of the predisposing genes develops Alzheimer's disease, and not having them is not an insurance against getting it. Clearly, there is a way to go before everything is understood about the relationship between the role of genes and Alzheimer's disease.

Further information on Alzheimer's

GUIDES TO RESEARCH, TREATMENT AND CARING

Alzheimer's: The Complete Guide for Families and Loved Ones, by Howard Gruetzner, John Wiley & Sons Inc., New York, 1997. (A small but comprehensive paperback covering the carer's experience, research and treatment options.)

The 'Research Briefs' section of *InTouch*, the quarterly journal for members of the Alzheimer's Association of NSW provides easy-to-read summaries of the latest research.

Useful sources can also be found on the internet. The Australian Alzheimer's Association web page is at www.alzheimers.org.au and the UK Alzheimer's Society also has a very informative web page, which can be found at www.alzheimers.org.uk

FIRST-HAND PERSPECTIVES OF PEOPLE WITH DAT

'Is it Dementia? Warning signs you should know', Alzheimer's Association NSW brochure, April 1997.

Who Will I be When I Die?, by Christine Boden, HarperCollins Religious, Melbourne, 1998.

Living in the Labyrinth, by Diana Friel McGowin, Thorndike Press audio by arrangement with Elder Books, 1993.

A CARER'S PERSPECTIVE

Early Stage Dementia: Reassurance for sufferers and carers, by Lorraine West, Hodder Headline Australia, Sydney, 2001.

Alzheimer's Disease: A Carer's Guide, by Bill Grant, Gore & Osment, Woollahra, 1993.

At a glance

- The term 'dementia' covers any loss of mental ability that impairs a person's ability to function independently. Alzheimer's disease is the most common form of dementia.

- The majority of people don't get Alzheimer's. Undue worry is caused by confusing incidence (the number of new cases per year) with prevalence (the total number of people with the disease).

- Differences between normal ageing and Alzheimer's occur in all areas of everyday functioning (thinking and reasoning, talking and listening, social and emotional abilities, movement and body control). In Alzheimer's the deterioration is persistent and progressive.

- Early treatment can slow the progression of Alzheimer's disease.

- Support, counselling and education are provided by family doctors, the Alzheimer's Association, and geriatric teams from public hospitals.

- Research continues into causes and treatment of dementia. Genes do play a role but it is thought that most forms of Alzheimer's are not inherited. Environmental factors (such as diet and lifestyle) that contribute to heart disease also seem to be risk factors for Alzheimer's.

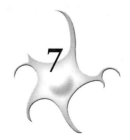

Maintaining Health for Vintage Memories

The three most important factors in
allowing us to live well for longer are
food variety, regular activity and being
socially active.[1]

Many people are willing to go to considerable lengths to improve their
memories but it is less well known which actions truly make a difference.
We all know good nutrition is important, but how good does it have to be?
And would supplements help further? We know exercise is beneficial, but is
gardening as good as a brisk walk? And would Tai Chi be better? Everyone
knows that a laugh feels good but does it just make us feel better, or do our
social lives materially affect our health?

Clear answers are now known for each of these questions. The role of
this chapter is to provide information on these and other major issues that
impact on memory, and the often avoidable substances and conditions that
may give short-term pleasure but long-term illness and poor health. Beliefs

determine attitudes and expectations, which in turn determine goals and drive actions. The more up-to-date information we have, the better. Providing our memories with the best possible care comes down to lifestyle choices.

Physical and social influences

Memory needs a brain, and a brain depends on the oxygen and glucose in the blood supply. A good blood supply needs a heart with muscles that can pump it around at sufficient force. The same blood also travels from the lungs through the brain's vascular system, carrying nutrients and oxygen and removing waste products. In fact, the brain takes a huge 20 per cent of the body's oxygen supply. Every action we take that enhances the health of heart, brain and blood supply (the cardiovascular system) will enhance the health of the memory system. Conversely, actions that damage cardiovascular health also damage memory.

The physical and social factors that enhance memory often depend on quite simple choices taken every day.

Exercise

> *I feel so alive and well when I come back from a walk I can hardly remember how difficult it was for me to get out of the house in the first place. There always seemed to be something else I needed to do first!*
> LOUISE (A FRIEND)

It is an agreeable surprise to many people to learn that the best thing they can do for memory is regular exercise like walking. Exercise is the key to getting more oxygen to the brain cells and providing optimum conditions for memory. In a remarkable study carried out by Arthur Kramer and his colleagues, two different types of exercise programs were investigated with the participation of 124 adults aged 60 to 75, who were not at the time exercising regularly.[2] For the study, half the group did stretching and toning exercises and the other half did energetic walking. After six months it was found that the walking group had improved memory for mental activities such as planning, scheduling and working memory, compared to the gentle exercise group.

Other studies have shown similar benefits of exercising. One of these studies recorded the physical activity (walking) of 5,925 women over six to eight years.[3] The average age of the women was 70 years. It was found that the most active of them (walking at least 1.6 kilometres per day) were the least likely to develop cognitive decline. The main reason given was increased blood flow to the brain, which reduces the risk of stroke and heart disease and stimulates the growth and survival of brain cells.

A desirable aim is to build up to 30 minutes of exercise on most days of the week. Walking should be brisk enough to feel puffed but still be able to hold a conversation. Increased heart rate should return to normal within five minutes of finishing exercise.[4] It takes about a month to accustom the body to a new habit so that the daily routine is accepted and welcomed.

Although any exercise is better than none, brisk walking is more effective than gardening because of the sustained workout for heart and lungs. If fear of falling puts a dampener on the wish to walk, exercises to improve balance and strengthen muscles have proven very effective in reducing the number of falls.[5] Appropriate exercise includes Tai Chi classes, consulting a physiotherapist, or home exercises, such as those described in Miriam Nelson's book, *Strong Women Stay Young*.[6]

For active exercise, precautions include:[7]

- See a doctor first to check blood pressure and any other risk factor.

- Drink plenty of fluids, particularly in warm weather.

- Wear well-fitting, flat-soled, non-slip shoes.

- Walk in a safe environment such as on level ground, when there is plenty of light and with at least one other person.

- Stop exercising if feeling unwell.

Sleep and memory[8]

> *Why after sleep or rest is memory often restored?*
> CHARLOTTE

Tiredness affects everyone's memory. Most people would agree from first-hand experience that lack of sleep causes difficulties with thinking and remembering.

Sleep has an obvious role in enhancing memory by countering tiredness, but it also plays several non-obvious roles in maintaining basic metabolic processes and repairing delicate brain structures. Sleep is also important for the long-term storage of memories because dreams are thought to be essential for the consolidation of memories.

Dreaming and deep sleep states alternate several times a night. The dreaming sleep states are characterised by rapid eye movement (REM) beneath closed eyelids, and sleepers lose all muscle tone and are difficult to wake. These periods are thought to play a crucial role in consolidating recently acquired memories. As we have seen in earlier chapters, a memory is actually a plethora of many different sights and sounds, bound up with times, places and feelings. The brain assembles recently acquired memories in a structure deep in the centre of the brain called the hippocampus. The multiple aspects of an episode are gradually integrated into the higher brain regions of the cortex for permanent storage over a period that may take years. Because of the nature of the long-term storage process, the transfer must be very slow or it could interfere with memories that have previously been stored. Dreams are thought to play a crucial role in this gradual transfer by repeatedly replaying very short fragments of events from recent days.[9]

People sometimes ask whether it would help the memory process if we tried to remember our dreams. The answer is probably not. If the theory about memory consolidation is accurate, then dreams are part of the regular housekeeping in the brain. When we remember one, it is like a brief glimpse of the hustle and bustle of the kitchen at a busy restaurant – interesting, but not something that we could contribute to in any meaningful way.

Learning something just before sleeping does seem to help retain it in memory better. During the last century there was a flurry of interest in learning *while* asleep with an audio tape playing. It was found to be quite ineffectual and there is no evidence that adults can learn anything while asleep. Intriguingly, it has recently been reported that new-born babies may learn simple sounds while asleep.[10]

DISTURBED SLEEP

Our sleeping and waking pattern – the circadian rhythm – is like a built-in clock regulated by several factors including exposure to sunlight and the hormone melatonin, which is released when it is dark.[11] The 24-hour cycle of sleeping and waking can become disturbed for a number of reasons, such as jet lag from changing time zones, shift work, winter depression, or any condition where people are wakeful through the night. The cycle can also be disturbed through illness or as people age and produce less melatonin.

Although older people tend to sleep less, regular and restful sleep is still important for maintaining a healthy and alert memory.

Many types of sleep disturbances can be helped by exposure to bright sunlight during the morning, or if that is not feasible, bright electric light will do. Five hours of bright light on each of three successive days can reset the internal clock by as much as 12 hours.[12] Exercise also improves the quality of sleep and walking in the morning can provide a useful adjunct.

Melatonin supplements are widely used by travellers to reset their internal clock and as a sleeping pill for people with low melatonin levels. Such supplements are not widely available in Australia, but are common in the USA and Europe. The evidence suggests that taking supplements is effective for some people, however self-medication is not recommended as melatonin regulates other brain hormones and the long-term effects of taking the hormone supplement are not known. Determining effective doses is complicated by the fact that people react very differently to melatonin supplements (even given the same dose), and doses in trials have varied widely from a fraction of a milligram to tens of milligrams. Richard Wurtman (a professor at the Massachusetts Institute of Technology and holder of a patent on the use of melatonin for controlling sleep) recommends that no more than 0.3 milligram should be taken to keep the hormone in the natural range, and this view is supported by sleep trials that have shown higher doses to be less effective than lower ones.[13]

Sleep problems can also be due to many other factors, including worry. One report in the *Oxford Handbook of Memory* estimates that in Western countries as many as '10 to 15 per cent of people over 65 years of age regularly take a type of sleeping pill that can induce a transient memory loss'.[14] When taken in combination with medications that act on the brain, they can cause confusion as well.

A variety of techniques can be used as alternatives to sleeping pills. Programs such as David Morawetz's *Sleep Better Without Drugs* (audio tape and booklet) provide information on a wide variety of common sleep problems and how to deal with them.[15] Sleeplessness due to a restless 'I must get to sleep' and repetition of busy thoughts is the result of an over-active left hemisphere in the brain.[16] As David Morawetz says, 'Most of the thinking and worrying that we do in bed needs to be done – it just does not need to be done in bed ... therefore make sure you devote some time each day to thinking and worrying, including thinking and worrying about not sleeping.'[17] It helps to review the previous day positively and count the successes rather than the downtimes, relegating difficulties to a mental shelf marked 'tomorrow'.

For people who have trouble falling asleep, audio tapes are often effective. Most commercial audio tapes have a calm voice that takes the listener through the relaxation techniques of lying down comfortably, drawing attention to various muscles that might be tense and concentrating on breathing. For example, a simple breathing exercise is to breathe in while counting to eight, holding the breath for four counts, then breathe out. After several cycles of breathing in this special way, let the mind wander over the whole body, moving arms and legs a little if needed to feel completely at rest and let the tension go.

Chronic sleep problems may require the attention of a specialist, and clinics can be consulted to deal with improving the quality of sleep. Major hospitals often have sleep disorder units.

Memory and social life

> *I am 88 years old, I drive, go out a lot, have lots of friends, hobbies, a dog, lots of fun and so far a happy life. I take my disabilities in my stride and try and keep my mind alert.*
> ZOE

Besides the traditional approaches to good health of exercise and rest, studies are finding that the complete picture also includes the effects of more intangible body needs, such as socialising and positive attitudes. Benefits occur as the result of a chain effect, with one thing affecting another which affects another. Thus warding off disease and keeping memory healthy is part of a chain that includes attitudes and behaviour arising from those attitudes.[18] Social life both uses and increases memory. Like love, the more you use the more you have.

People who participate in several social domains, such as family, friends, work, and other groups, have a variety of health benefits. They include better survival from heart attacks, lower recurrence of cancer and less depression than their more isolated counterparts. The benefits even include a lower chance of catching the common cold.[19] Studies in Finland, Sweden and the United States have all shown that loneliness and social isolation can have a devastating effect on those who feel they have no one to rely upon or in whom to confide their innermost thoughts and feelings.[20] To cope with stress in their lives, people need a support group or even just one staunch friend (who could, of course, be a spouse or relative). The support can vary in how much, how often and what form it takes, but the essential factor is that there is someone who values and cares for us and could be relied upon to give help in times of crisis.

Positive attitudes also have demonstrated links to good health. For example, the Ohio Longitudinal Study of Aging and Retirement studied how positive and negative attitudes to ageing influenced people's lives.[21] The study included 660 people aged 50 to 94 and was conducted over 23 years. Self-perceptions were rated on each person's view of their life as full or empty, hopeful or hopeless, and worthy or worthless. It found that the people who had a positive attitude to their life lived on average seven and a half years longer than those who had a more negative attitude. The figure stands even after taking into account age, gender, socio-economic status, loneliness and functional health. That is to say, the people who lived longest were not necessarily the ones blessed with the best health, friends and income, but they were the ones who had achieved a positive attitude to their own ageing.

> *People need people. Be a joiner. Try to get to know a few younger people. Have lots of walks. Eat the right food – lots of veg and fruit and a little red meat etc. Do some relaxation exercise. Work for a charity. I think some people are overly concerned about memory loss – it happens when you are young.*
> ALI

Nutrition and supplements

Traditionally, children have been told 'Eat your greens, they're good for you'. But we all know people who don't eat sensibly and seem (at least superficially) to be coping okay. One extreme stereotype is the person who survives on pizza, chips and soft drink. Are youngsters with poor diet storing up problems for much later in life? How much of a difference does good nutrition really make to memory in the short and the long term?

From day to day, memory depends on adequate calories and avoiding excessive negative influences. Research has shown that older people are better at remembering after they have eaten breakfast than when they are hungry, and in general, need to eat smaller meals more often to function at peak performance.[22]

In the longer term, good memory depends on the type of food eaten. Some long-term influences are well documented, such as the benefits of vegetables and exercise on all aspects of health or the negative effects of saturated fats and excessive salt on heart disease. The evidence for a wide variety of other factors such as supplements and alternative medicines is still being collected and evaluated. Major studies of different eating habits and the health of the participants have led nutritionists to revise their advice on healthy eating and the structure of healthy-eating pyramids.

Nutrients not just calories

> *Sham Harga had run a successful eatery for many years by always smiling, never extending credit, and realizing that most of his customers wanted meals properly balanced between the four food groups: sugar, starch, grease and burnt crunchy bits.*
> TERRY PRATCHETT[23]

'Diet' is what we eat in our normal (and often abnormal) lifestyles, and includes supplements of any kind, including alternative medicines and indulgence foods. How do we know when we have an adequate diet? Vitamins and minerals have no detectable taste, so we need other ways to ensure our diet is balanced.

In general, a lifestyle of healthy and tasty eating habits means eating a wide variety of foods and including all food groups. Within food groups, variety is also necessary. The nutritionists Gayle Savige, Mark Wahlqvist and their colleagues advise eating at least 20 biologically distinct foods per week (including fruits, vegetables, grains, nuts, meats, diary, fish, eggs, oils, herbs and spices).[24]

Most people are aware of a connection between cholesterol and heart disease. Cholesterol is a form of fat that is needed to make hormones and is a component of cell membranes. The body makes its own cholesterol as well as storing the oversupply eaten in food. What is important for health is the ratio of the two main cholesterol-carrying chemicals, popularly known as 'bad cholesterol' (LDL) and 'good cholesterol' (HDL). The maximum benefit seems to be gained by replacing saturated fat (found mainly in animal foods such as fatty meat, butter and cream and a few plants such as coconut and palm oils) with unsaturated fat, including monounsaturated fats (found in olive and canola oil, most nuts and avocadoes) and omega-3 fatty acids (a type of polyunsaturated fat found in canola, linseed, walnuts, soybeans, fish and green vegetables).[25]

Until the 1990s, it was generally recommended that most calories in a healthy diet should come from carbohydrates, rather than fats and oils. More recently, epidemiological and nutrition studies have shown that not all carbohydrates are good for us, just as not all fats and oils are bad.[26] Carbohydrates in the form of whole grains are complex carbohydrates and are generally beneficial for health. Refined carbohydrates (such as white bread and white rice) and those that are mostly starch (like white potatoes) are very different and act like refined sugar in that they can be too quickly broken down into glucose.[27] As the body tries to control the glucose levels with increased production of insulin, the initial peak can be followed by a rapid drop in blood sugar. Associated feelings of tiredness can stimulate a person to eat more and repeat the cycle again. Professors of epidemiology and nutrition at the Harvard School of Public Health, Walter Willett and Meir Stampfer, have lamented that 'Unfortunately, many nutritionists decided that it would be too difficult to educate the public about these subtleties'.[28] Willet and Stampfer take up the challenge and explain the issues in their comprehensive article in the January 2003 edition of *Scientific American*.

Over the years, many different organisations have developed healthy eating plans, based on the best advice available and the needs of the community at the time. In times of war and shortages the need is to ensure that the population is adequately fed. In affluent times, the need is to restrict indulgence foods and balance the calories appropriately across the food groups. People who are overweight and inactive and have diets high in refined carbohydrates have much higher risks of heart disease and diabetes, so much current advice about healthy eating focusses on weight reduction and balancing cholesterol levels.

Willett and Stampfer recommend a revised food pyramid in which both wholegrain foods and plant oils (olive, canola, soy, corn, sunflower, peanut and other vegetable oils) are eaten at most meals. Vegetables should be eaten in abundance, with two to three servings of fruit per day. They also suggest one to three servings of nuts and legumes, up to two servings of fish, poultry or eggs, one serving of dairy or a calcium supplement, and sparing intake of red meat, butter, white rice, white bread, potatoes, pasta and sweets.[29] They report that replacing some carbohydrates and proteins by the same number of calories in nuts and oils can be more satisfying to the appetite and lower the risk of heart disease and diabetes. The idea is to keep the overall total calories down, not just calories from fat. They also stress the importance of exercise as the foundation of their food pyramid, since the number of calories we eat should be balanced against the exercise we do. (These guidelines are illustrated in the pyramid diagram below.)

Many variations on the food pyramid have been devised. If red meat (beef, lamb and pork) is included in any food plan, lean meat is always recommended. However, the recommended amounts vary widely and individuals should consider their own particular needs. A 1992 CSIRO plan called '12345+' proposed small amounts of lean red meat on most days to ensure an adequate supply of iron and zinc.[30] Vegetarian diets recommend other sources of protein, including nuts and legumes.

Many food plans sensibly include a place – a very small place – for indulgence foods such as cakes, biscuits, sweets, pastries, pies, soft drinks and alcohol (unless there are contraindications).

All the plans we looked at agreed on the importance of vegetables and fruits, and eating a wide variety of food types. Many other aspects of diet merit attention and many excellent up-to-date sources can be consulted for a more complete treatment.[31]

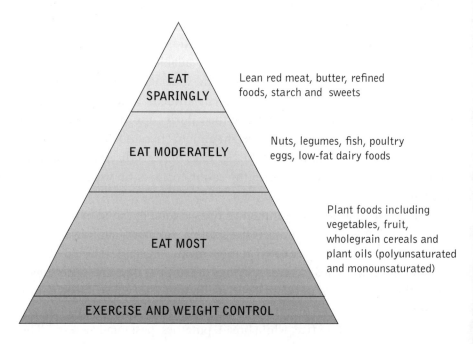

The three tiers of the healthy eating pyramid is built on a base
of exercise and weight control.[32]

Vitamins

Which vitamins/chemical substances would improve retention of memory in later life? – prevention being important.
CHRIS

Vitamins play a special role in maintaining health and memory. Vitamins are nutrients made up of more than one ingredient (organic compound).[33] There are 13 vitamins (at last count) and most have many sub-groups. They were discovered and analysed in the 1930s and 1940s but since then there has been some shuffling and re-numbering. All the vitamins are essential because they have different services to perform for the body. They work in close cooperation with companion nutrients found in cereals, nuts, legumes, fruit and vegetables. Their companion nutrients include hundreds of plant chemicals, called phytochemicals (phyto is Greek for plant).[34] For example, the vitamin beta carotene (one of the A group) is normally found in foods in companionship with about 600 related substances. Interactions between vitamins and phytochemicals are essential for their utilisation by the body.

Vitamins are absorbed differently depending on whether they are soluble in fat or water. Water-soluble ones include the vitamin B group and vitamin C and must be eaten often, since an over-supply is excreted in urine. Fat-soluble vitamins (A, D, E, and K) are absorbed better if eaten with fats or oils. They are stored by the body (mainly in the liver) so an excess can be hazardous to health. In a normal balanced diet it would be difficult to have too much of any one vitamin. A more common problem is likely to be a lack of essential phytochemicals due to eating too narrow a range of foods.

A ground-swell of research over the past ten years has shown that correcting subtle nutritional deficiencies by eating sufficient amount of fruits and vegetables and taking some supplements can prevent or slow the development of diseases (in the elderly).
WORLD HEALTH ORGANISATION[35]

Antioxidants for protection

Oxygen is familiar to us as part of the air we breathe. It is necessary for normal body metabolism but as a by-product it also produces particles called free radicals. These particles play important roles such as fighting infection, however, in excessive numbers they become harmful and damage the lipids (fats), carbohydrates and proteins that comprise the body's cells, including the oily walls of brain cells. They can also damage DNA, the chemical code from which genes are constructed and such damage is now thought to play an important role in ageing.[36] Free radicals can be neutralised by antioxidants, a class of substances that prevent oxidation and can significantly delay or prevent many types of damage such as happens with cardiovascular disease and cognitive decline.

The body has an army of substances that work as antioxidants. There are literally thousands of them, found in a wide variety of foods or produced by the body (endogenous enzymes). The main nutritional antioxidants are the vitamins A, C, and E and hundreds of phytochemicals. These include the carotenoids (named for the red, yellow and orange pigments found in plants), the flavonoids (found in the skin of grapes, red wine, tea, apples and citrus), and polyphenols (found in cranberries, raspberries and blackberries and the herbs rosemary, oregano and thyme).[37] Other antioxidants include the hormones oestrogen and melatonin, the minerals selenium and zinc, the co-enzyme Q10 (found in oily fish, lean meat, soy beans, nuts and oils and essential for metabolism) and aspirin (best known as a pain killer and anti-inflammatory medication).

When to take supplements

The additions we can make to our diets in pill form are numerous and can be good, bad or indifferent in terms of health and memory.[38] Supplements do not generally target memory performance directly, but rather target general improvements in cardiovascular health. They can reduce cholesterol, scavenge free radicals through additional antioxidants, and increase attention and alertness by dilating blood vessels, which can increase the effectiveness of brain cells through increased supplies of oxygen and glucose.

Given a consistently healthy diet, supplements of antioxidants or vitamins should not be necessary, particularly for young to middle-aged individuals. Healthy older people do not necessarily need supplements, although they are frequently less active and need fewer calories, and therefore need to be more aware of the nutritional value of the food they do eat.[39] However, many of us are aware that our diets are not always as good as they could be. In fact, it has been estimated that less than 10 per cent of Australians eat a consistently balanced diet.[40] As the psychologist John Pinel notes, 'Even rats prefer chocolate chip cookies to nutritionally complete rat chow.'[41]

Reasons for considering supplements might be known risks such as high cholesterol, diabetes, shortages in the diet or preventative measures against degenerative diseases.

Taking supplements is somewhat like buying an insurance policy to protect your most valuable asset (your health) for the future. The general advice of 'buyer beware' holds: make sure you're insuring the right thing, know what you're buying and read the fine print. However, unlike insurance, which is only an expensive waste if you don't need it, levels of vitamins or hormones that are too high could actively damage the very systems you are trying to protect, or damage others that are currently functioning well. One worthwhile investment is a small book on vitamins (such as *Vitamins* by Rosemary Stanton).[42]

The main kinds of commercial supplements offered for memory are vitamin and mineral tablets, other plant-based substances such as gingko biloba, and medication added to foods (for example, cholesterol-lowering substances added to margarines). Choosing which if any of these three areas to add to one's diet can be confusing for the individual, and much additional clinical research is required before their safety and effective doses are well understood and agreed on by nutritionists.

We briefly summarise relevant issues for each of these areas in the following pages, and recommend that readers consult their health advisers to tailor a program for their individual needs, taking into account such factors as health, fitness level, weight, age and gender.

SUPPLEMENTS FOR ANTIOXIDANTS

The best recommendation for an adequate supply of antioxidants each day is:

vegetables	3 servings (1 cup)
fruit	2 pieces

Of course, fresh food is not generally considered a 'supplement', but for some people's diets it should be! On days when a shortfall in fruit and vegetables occurs, many health researchers consider that supplements of antioxidants are generally considered safe and may have health benefits. Jeff Coombes, a researcher into antioxidants and ageing, recommends top-ups of:[43]

vitamin C	500 milligrams per day
vitamin E	400 milligrams per day.

Excess vitamin C is eliminated from the body, but very high doses can stress the kidneys. Vitamin E is fat soluble, so excess amounts can build up in the body and it is toxic in large quantities (amounts under 1,000 milligrams per day are generally considered safe but maximum levels for different body weights have not been determined).[44] Supplements of vitamin E should not be taken in the weeks immediately before or after surgery because it reduces the ability of the blood to clot and can cause internal bleeding. The suggested dosages are for an average-sized person and individuals should discuss an appropriate dose for themselves with their health adviser. Note that too high a dose of any substance that acts as an antioxidant may act as a pro-oxidant and be potentially harmful to other body processes.[45] Vitamin A is also a potent antioxidant and supplements are sometimes recommended as part of an antioxidant top-up, however the amount should not exceed 5 milligrams per day (equivalent to one small carrot) since recent studies have shown increased risk of cancer from the supplement form of vitamin A but not from natural foods.[46]

Note that supplements should not be used as a sole source of vitamins and minerals as they lack the wealth of companion nutrients that are found in fruit and vegetables, which may be necessary for their work as antioxidants to be effective.[47]

GINGKO BILOBA AND OTHER ALTERNATIVE REMEDIES

I would like to see research on alternative medication, i.e. vitamins, minerals, Western and Chinese herbs, on the memory.
VENETIA

Alternative remedies are called 'alternative' as they use substances that are purported to have therapeutic value but have not been tested via the usual clinical trials for medicines. Alternative medicines originate from a wide variety of sources, including many from non-Western countries, where some have been used for centuries. There is comparatively little scientific research on alternative medicines because most such research is funded by commercial interests. As *Choice* magazine notes, 'Herbs cannot be patented, so there is little financial incentive for companies to make the investment.'[48] There is, therefore, a difficulty in assessing their efficacy, and a lack of standardisation compared to conventional medicines.

Many substances are known for their power to briefly enhance memory by countering fatigue, boosting arousal, or increasing circulation and alertness. These include caffeine, aspirin, vitamin E and oestrogen. Evidence suggests that the normal human brain usually runs as well as it can and little additional improvement is possible.[49] As the neuroscientists Larry Squire and Eric Kandel comment, 'the issue is no longer whether in normal aging some treatment can improve the score on a memory test, but whether memory can be improved beyond what one can do with a good cup of coffee.'[50]

One substance that has been frequently in the news and has been assessed in a variety of studies is gingko biloba extract, which has been used for centuries in Chinese medicine. The ginkgo biloba (maiden hair) tree is an ancient form of conifer from Asia. Its leaves are used to make the extract that is widely thought to enhance memory. It is sold in Australia without prescription, as a pill under different brand names. The active ingredient is called ginko biloba extract, or GBE, and is provided in differing amounts in different products. The exact role of ginko biloba extract is not clearly understood, but the benefits are generally thought to include improved blood flow to the brain, which provides increases in oxygen and nutrients. It is also an antioxidant, and hence may assist in preventing cell damage.

Over the past 25 years, many studies have tested the effects of GBE in treating cognitive decline.[51] In severe dementias, such as vascular dementia and Alzheimer's, one study showed that improvements in symptoms lasted from six to 12 months. In cases of mild memory loss, it has sometimes provided improvement and helped reduce stress in older people, in one case with benefits most obvious after four weeks of treatment.

GBE is also taken as a short-term memory booster by people with no clinically observable cognitive decline. Quantifying the benefits has been difficult, since doses are not standardised and different studies use different amounts, however, there seems to be consensus that it may assist in tasks involving working memory, but has less or no effect on arousal or selective attention. The optimum dose for improved performance is also uncertain. In fact, in a study that compared performance for different doses, the lowest dose was more beneficial than higher ones.[52]

Overall, studies show that GBE may have small beneficial effects for some people with dementia or mild memory loss, but benefit for others has not been established. As with other stimulants, high doses should be avoided as GBE can cause heart dysrhythmia and it should not be taken in conjunction with aspirin (nor any other additive that reduces blood clotting) as it can cause internal bleeding.

FOOD AS MEDICATION

Over past decades, additions to food and drink have been made for the health of the community, such as fluoride in water to prevent dental decay, and the vitamin thiamin in bread. These additives were made on government initiative, rather than driven by commercial interests.[53] At present there is little Australian government funding for food research and many food scientists now work for commercial interests.[54] Currently, the drive to put medications in foods is coming from the large food companies whose need to be profitable leads them to constantly seek new markets. Supermarket shelves are stocking foods with medication added, such as margarine with added cholesterol-lowering substances. Such 'doctored' foods have been given the name of 'functional foods', or sometimes 'nutriceuticals' or 'smart foods'.[55]

Medicated foods should be treated as medicines, and discussed with your health adviser to consider their role in a complete treatment program. One early concern was that additives to reduce cholesterol may also reduce the beneficial effects of the carotenoids (vitamin A). If an enriched margarine or other dairy product is eaten, an extra daily intake of yellow vegetables may be needed to offset possible losses.[56] Another concern is that children or pregnant women may accidentally eat the enriched products with detrimental effects. As with supplements and alternative medicines, the take-home message of medicated foods is to be clear about what is being taken and why.

Caveat emptor

When considering supplements, simple precautions to guard against ill effects include:

- Learn about the body's requirements for vitamins, the best sources from natural foods, and why (or if) each supplement is needed.[57] Don't be misled by unrealistic hype.

- Be sensibly cautious with all medicines and health additives. Read labels to know what is in the product, the recommended dose and how much of each active ingredient is in it. Words such as 'light' or 'lite' may only refer to colour; and 'no cholesterol' does not mean there are no other fats. Characterising ingredients must be listed but the catch is the definition of 'characterising'. For example, in wholemeal bread, the amount of wholemeal in the flour is not considered characterising.[58]

- Inform health advisers of all supplements being taken. Both herbal additives and conventional medicines can have side-effects, particularly when taken with other medications, just before surgery, or in overdose quantities.[59]

Government regulations

We are so used to government regulation of food and medicines in general that there is a tendency to assume that supplements would not be available unless they are safe. In fact this is not the case, and health products have different levels of regulation.[60] Many substances sold as health additives have not been quality tested and their claims may not have been substantiated. Alternative medicines are not standardised and there can be differences between brands or batches of the same brand in terms of the quality and quantity of the ingredients.[61]

The sale of food is regulated by the Food Standards Australia and New Zealand (FSANZ, previously the Australia and New Zealand Food Authority).[62] Novel foods, genetically modified and irradiated food, as well as any new additives or changes within those already on the market require the approval of FSANZ. Labels for food must give:

- A name for the food.

- A list of ingredients and percentage of characterising ingredients.

- A 'use by' or 'best before' date.

- A nutrition information panel.

- The name and address in Australia of the manufacturer.

There is an international seal of approval called G.R.A.S. (Generally Regarded As Safe) for foods such as potatoes, rice and oranges that have been used by large numbers of people for hundreds of years. If a product has passed set nutrition criteria the tick of the Heart Foundation may be used. However, because there is a fee to be paid, not all manufacturers apply for the tick for their eligible products.

Medicines are regulated by the Therapeutic Goods Association. New conventional medicines, obtainable by prescription from doctors, must be tested and approved by clinical trials. Herbal medicines can be either voluntarily listed or registered with the Therapeutic Goods Administration. Ones that are listed have 'Australian L' marked on the label, which denotes that the substance is low risk and makes modest claims. If registered 'Australian R' with a registration number on the label, the product has also been tested for safety, quality and efficacy.[63]

Risks and hazards

Major hazards to memory (and life in general) include cardiovascular disease and addictive substances and we can try and minimise their worst affects. We can't change our family history, age or sex, but there are several factors that are under our control. The major ones are smoking, raised blood cholesterol levels, high blood pressure, physical inactivity and being overweight.

Body Mass Index (BMI)

The Body Mass Index (BMI) is a way of indicating if a person's weight is within acceptable limits for good health. To calculate the index use the following method:

Method	Example
1 Measure weight in kilograms	80 kilograms
2 Measure height in metres	1.7 metres
3 Square the height	1.7 x 1.7 = 2.89
4 Divide weight by height squared	80 / 2.89 = 28

The example person is 1.7m (5'7") tall, weighs 80kg and their BMI is 28. The upper index for a healthy weight is 25 (and more than 30 is considered obese), so this person is overweight. For their height, they should aim for a maximum weight of 72kg.[64] Every one degree decrease in BMI decreases the risk of stroke by 6 per cent.[65]

Cardiovascular disease

Does heart disease have any bearing on memory loss? I feel bad circulation has some impact – is this correct?

THELMA

Cardiovascular diseases are those of the heart and blood vessels. Impeded or diminished blood supply caused by narrowing and clogging of blood vessels can cause heart attacks and strokes. Clogging is caused by plaques on the inside of blood vessels from fatty deposits such as cholesterol. When the brain has reduced blood supply, memory is affected.

In the last 50 years the rate of heart attacks has halved as a result of changes people have made in their lifestyles and improved medical treatment. The welcome reduction, particularly for men, is due in part to the work of the Heart Foundation and the successful public health campaign advising on the unhealthy effects of animal fats in the diet and problems of being overweight, which influence blood pressure levels and blood cholesterol levels. However, heart disease is still the leading cause of disability and death in Australia.[66]

Damaging substances

The substance nicotine in cigarette smoke causes the release of acetylcholine, a neurotransmitter (a chemical messenger in the brain) increasing alertness and memory in the short-term. Nicotine also activates the neurotransmitter dopamine to bind to cells in the brain's reward pathways, causing a feeling of pleasure. But the effect soon wears off. In the longer term, smoking in later life (over 65 years) seems to be linked to added risk of intellectual impairment. Researchers found that smokers were up to four times more likely to have evidence of significant intellectual decline than either non-smokers or former smokers.[67] The main trouble is that the red blood cells can carry less oxygen to the brain because the space has been usurped by the carbon monoxide in cigarette smoke. Non-smokers in the same room are affected as well. 'After quitting, the body can rid itself of nicotine and carbon monoxide within twelve hours and nicotine by-products within a few days. Blood flow to the limbs improves within two months and lungs regain the capacity to clean themselves within three months.'[68]

No one, least of all smokers, has a good word to say about smoking. As everyone knows, the problem is that it is highly addictive. Some hospitals and community health centres run courses for giving up smoking, covering aspects like how to beat cravings, how to handle withdrawal, and how to stay stopped. There are useful books on the market on how to plan for and give up smoking as well as the Quitline phone service (phone 131848). The website www.quitnow.info.au also has useful information.

Alcohol used to be equally paired with smoking as a health hazard but more recently moderate drinking of alcohol has been found not to be detrimental to health and even beneficial in some circumstances.[69] Red wine is often mentioned as being an antioxidant but it has a very small amount compared to some of the vitamins. A moderate number of drinks per day is no more than two for men and one for women, with some alcohol-free days each week.[70]

Alcohol first causes arousal, followed by decreased alertness. The pleasure of drinking is due to its dampening effect on a particular neurotransmitter called GABA. Medication treatment for excessive drinking targets the GABA neurons, thus reducing the pleasure of drinking and effectively reducing the desire for alcohol.[71]

Excessive drinking increases the risk of health problems, in particular high blood pressure, heart disease and stroke. Combined with poor diet over a long period it can also lead to a catastrophic breakdown in mental ability.[72]

Anaesthesia

> [I would like to know about] the effects of
> anaesthesia on memory.
> VENETIA

Anaesthesia is the medical use of special chemicals to induce unconsciousness. General anaesthetics appear to work by targeting a region of the brain thought to control general awareness and arousal.[73] The chemicals of the anaesthetic insert themselves within cell membranes so that they disrupt the cells' normal functioning, preventing the cells from sending and receiving messages. The exact mechanism is not known, although it is thought that they interact with either the lipids or proteins of the cell membrane.

Anaesthetics have improved markedly over the last 20 years. A common practice now is for the anaesthetist to prepare a 'cocktail' of ingredients suited to the patient and the surgical procedure. Such a cocktail could include a muscle relaxant, an analgesic for pain relief and an anaesthetic agent to induce temporary memory loss. Such a cocktail ensures that the patient won't remember the operation but will have similar memory abilities to before the anaesthetic. Light anaesthesia can cause post-operative drowsiness and memory loss for a day or two, which then wears off completely. Major surgery (such as that needed for heart bypass surgery) can affect memory for a longer period, even several months, but such memory loss is generally thought to be due to the associated illness and not the anaesthetic.

Depression

One reversible cause of memory loss is depression.[74] Depression is an identifiable illness which needs medical treatment. Its core feature is a dulling of emotion. It is not just an expression like sadness or loneliness, although depressed people do feel sad and they find decision making and concentrating difficult. The person feels numb – some people say that everything looks grey and negative. It can be associated with physical symptoms such as insomnia and lack of appetite.

The causes of depression are not known, but predisposing factors include genetics, stress, certain personality traits and diet.[75] Stressful trigger factors include losing a job, fatigue, grief, an overload of information, or even a belief that mental or physical decline is inevitable. Lack of well-being is an important contributor to depression in older ages, and people who feel well and have coping strategies to handle their problems suffer less from depression.[76]

Several neurotransmitters (chemical messengers in the brain) play a role in mood. Serotonin is one that plays an important role in memory and is low in people with depression. Several types of treatments address the physical basis of depression by boosting the effect of serotonin. Such direct targeting of serotonin levels involves medications such as the common antidepressant Prozac. An adequate diet is also important for treating people with depression, since the body requires specific proteins to make serotonin.

Alternatively, serotonin levels can be raised by addressing the psychological basis of depression. Cognitive therapy is one such approach that doesn't use medications but involves talking through problems to place them in a different perspective and developing coping skills.[77] Memory returns to normal when the depression is treated.

Stress and the immune system[78]

I believe that when I am stressed I tend to forget more.
DIANA

Stress is tension or strain and can be mental, emotional, or physical.[79] It activates the sympathetic nervous system which prepares the body for 'fight or flight' by increasing heart rate and blood pressure and slowing digestion.[80] When the stressful event is over, the parasympathetic system effects the opposite, thereby conserving the body's energy resources.

Stress is stress but some is more so than others. Short bursts of stress can be beneficial but long-term, uncontrolled stress can have serious effects on health. Good stress includes short-term events, such as moderate exercise, which can enhance the immune system.[81] In such cases, the initial stress response appears to prepare the body to fight infections, mobilise energy responses and inhibit inflammation.[82]

One-off events lasting minutes to hours (such as an exam or public speaking) appear to exacerbate allergies such as asthma, and inflammatory diseases such as rheumatoid arthritis. Bad stress is chronic, repeated or physiologically exhausting stress. Chronic stress persists for periods of several hours over many days or months and can result from bereavement, long-term illness or caring for a person with dementia. It appears to suppress immunity and increase susceptibility to infections and cancer.

> *Obviously, the immune system does not 'know' that a feared examination is at hand, that a spouse has died, or that social support is available. But the brain knows, and there is increasing evidence that what the brain knows and does can affect how well the immune system protects us.*[83]

Individual responses to stressful events can differ markedly.[84] The same life events can be perceived by one person as extremely stressful, but only mildly so by another (for example, public speaking). What someone feels about an event determines which stress-related emotions are experienced, including anxiety, anger, guilt, sadness, shame, envy and disgust.[85] In addition, how much control a person feels they have over the situation, their coping skills and the available social support also contribute to the stress reaction. For example, losing a job is stressful for everyone, but it is likely to be even more so for someone who has little social support.[86]

Everyone faces stress from different events and a range of coping strategies is useful. Being problem-focussed is one type of coping strategy, which involves making active attempts to confront and directly deal with the situation, such as seeking extra help if caring for a sick person. A second type of strategy is emotion focussed, where a person aims to assess and manage their own stress levels, such as using a relaxation tape to control tension. A third approach involves turning to other people for both assistance and emotional support.[87] Factors that can help to reduce the stress for other people include helping them to feel they have increased control over their lives and providing social support.

> *The greatest discovery of my generation is that a human being can alter his life by altering his attitude.*
> WILLIAM JAMES (FATHER OF PSYCHOLOGY)[88]

At a glance

- Exercise is important for getting more oxygen to the brain cells and providing optimum conditions for memory.

- Sleep enhances memory by facilitating brain maintenance, and consolidating newly acquired memories during dreaming sleep. Relaxation techniques can release tension before sleep.

- Social support is necessary for optimum health.

- Eat a wide variety of foods each week with abundant vegetables and fruit, wholegrains and some unsaturated oils.

- Antioxidants such as vitamins E, C and A are essential to deal with damaging free radicals. Supplements in pill form may be helpful if the daily intake of fresh food falls short.

- Read labels to be aware of what you are buying. Inform health advisers of supplements/medications taken to avoid clashes with medications.

- Major risk factors for cardiovascular disease include smoking, high cholesterol levels, high blood pressure, physical inactivity and being overweight.

- Avenues of help for smoking and excessive alcohol consumption include hospital clinics and community health centres, books on how to quit and the phone service Quitline.

- Depression and stress are reversible causes of memory loss and with treatment, memory can return to normal.

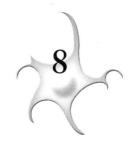

8

The Brain in Action

> To a first approximation, the overall function of the
> brain is to be well informed about what goes on in the
> rest of the body, ... what goes on in itself; and about the
> environment surrounding the organism ...[1]

Scientists had mapped the craters on the moon decades before they mapped
the regions of the brain. Studying this well-hidden control tower of brain
tissue has been difficult for several reasons. Early mappers of the brain first
had to name what they found without the advantage of knowing what each
part of the brain did. In every field early explorers latch on to whatever
similarities they can find. Brain parts were named for what they looked
like or the position in the brain of the structures, dignified by the Latin (or
Greek, French or English) translation. Thus we have the:

- hippocampus – Greek for sea monster, because of its curved shape

- cortex – Latin for husk, because it looks like wrinkled bark

- dendrite – Greek for tree, because of all its branches

- amygdala – Old English for almond, because of its shape
- glial – Greek for glue, the role first attributed to these cells.

The appearance of the brain gives us no inkling of the astounding performance of which it is capable and what an amazing powerhouse it really is. We can only appreciate the brain's staggering complexity in the living, functioning person and this has finally been possible in the last decade or so since technology has improved brain imaging. Electron microscopes enable scientists to look at the tiny cells of the brain and ingenious staining techniques allow them to trace the intricate networks formed by the cells and their long connections. We no longer need to think of the brain as a black box into which we cannot peer.

There have been various attempts to estimate the brain's capacity for storing knowledge.[2] One such method was to assume that the brain can process one bit of information per second by reading, so if we multiply the number of seconds in a lifetime by the number of neurons in the brain, we end up with totally unmanageable and meaningless figures! Present-day thinking is that a healthy brain's capacity to learn is limited only by attention, fatigue, mood and stress.

We can't have a good memory, or any memory, without a brain. How can such a head full of proteins and lipids and carbohydrates sparkle with thoughts and plans that can send a space probe to Jupiter, write the Declaration of Human Rights or share a laugh with friends? In this chapter we take a quick tour of some aspects that brain sciences have uncovered, tracing how our amazing brains organise and coordinate memories.

Physical characteristics[3]

The brain weighs about 1.25 kilograms in an average adult and is soft and floppy beneath its protective bony skull. The difference in the size of brains between adults has no influence on how intelligent they are. (Einstein, one of the greatest thinkers of the 20th century, did not have a big head.) The power of memory is based on the intricate connections between the nerve cells, not just how many cells there are.

The brain is a walnut-shaped organ, with two halves or hemispheres joined in the middle by a thick band of nerve fibres called the corpus callosum. Under the hemispheres are the cerebellum and the brain stem, which continues down through the base of the skull to become the spinal cord. Cerebellum and brain stem are both parts of what is called the 'old brain' (old in evolutionary terms), concerned with basic bodily functions such as control of breathing, sleeping and waking.

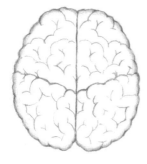

A top view of the walnut-shaped brain, showing the two halves or hemispheres. They are joined lower down by a thick band of fibres, the corpus callosum.

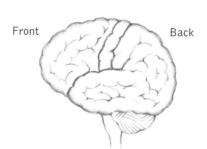

Front   Back

A left-side view of the brain showing the cerebellum and spinal cord.

Like the bark of a tree, the surface of the brain is wrinkled and convoluted, packed as it is into a space too small for it. If it was stretched out, it would be the size of a tea towel.[4] Called the cerebral cortex, it is a mere 2 millimetres thick, packed tight with the microscopic cell bodies which give a pinky-grey colour to the brain surface. Underneath the cortex is the tightly packed whitish brain matter of projections reaching from the cortex to other cells.

Cell types[5]

The brain is packed full of cells of a hundred different types. A hundred billion of these cells are neurons, which are the hub of the brain's processing power. They come in a huge variety of shapes and sizes, but generally consist of a cell body with a nucleus, many tentacle-like structures called dendrites, which receive signals from other cells, and a longish projection called an axon, which conveys signals to other neurons.

Less well known than neurons are a second kind of brain cell found in vast numbers – a thousand billion of them, ten times more than the number of neurons in the brain! Smaller than neurons, they are called glial cells and they have an important function in protecting and grooming the neurons, carrying nutrients to and waste materials from them and removing dead cells.[6] They produce an important substance called myelin that insulates the neurons and facilitates their work. The sheathing process is largely complete by the age of eight and finally complete by the age of 25.

The blood-brain barrier: the cell wall

The brain is included in the body's vascular system, with tiny capillaries networking around the neurons. Each neuron is well protected by an oily double membrane composed of the fats cholesterol and lecithin. Within the wall are various proteins which transport nutrients and oxygen from the capillary blood vessel through the wall to the cell nucleus.[7] This wall is the 'blood-brain barrier' and is very selective about which substances it will let pass through, even excluding potentially helpful medications. As one commentator quipped, taking supplements to help brain cells is like trying to help a country with acute fuel shortage by flying over the land and tipping cans of petrol over it.

Proteins[8]

The word 'protein' is familiar to us as a class of food, but it is the very stuff of life in us too. Proteins are constructed of amino acids (which come in 20 basic forms) in very many different configurations. There are countless numbers of proteins, each with a different function. They make up the walls of the cells; they act as enzymes (an enzyme is a catalyst which induces changes in other substances); and they are neurotransmitters, the brain's chemical messengers.

Proteins come in all sizes. For example, peptides are very small proteins, and some function as neuromodulators, which are chemical transmitters that adjust the sensitivity of cells to other neurotransmitters, such as in pain modulation.[9] Other proteins are very large, such as glycoproteins, which are embedded on the outer surface of a cell membrane at the synaptic gap between two neurons, ready to receive incoming messages from the neighbouring cell. It is thought that glycoproteins assist in the chain of events needed to turn short-term memories into long-term ones.

Genes and chromosomes[10]

Each neuron carries with it a complete set of instructions for making the proteins that it needs (as do all other cells). A new protein is constructed by

The Lego® factory[11]

Imagine a factory that takes Lego® blocks and assembles them into cars, household appliances, factory components, building materials, in fact everything needed for a Lego® society. This factory has one hundred thousand plans, one for each of the things it builds, including plans for all its own machines and Lego® robot workers, so it can repair its machines and build new ones when needed. It can even make a complete replica of the factory itself. The amazing thing about this factory is that it is built almost entirely out of Lego® blocks plus some simple components that are delivered to its door.

Cells are like factories that make proteins. Simple Lego® pieces correspond to amino acids (the building blocks of proteins), plans correspond to genes, and the assembled structures correspond to proteins that are needed to run the body.

stringing together amino acids like beads on a string, so the instructions for a protein need only provide the appropriate sequence of amino acids. Genes are such instructions.

Genes are coded in long threadlike molecules which we know as DNA (deoxyribonucleic acid). Humans have 23 pairs of DNA molecules (the chromosomes), which are arranged in double-stranded spirals. The chromosomes are coiled and packed into the nucleus of the cell.

To reproduce proteins essential for the life of the cell, the DNA molecule uncoils, the appropriate gene turns on (which just means that its instructions are copied) and then the DNA recoils again. The copy of the instructions is taken outside the nucleus to structures that string together the appropriate sequence of amino acids and fold the string into a protein.

Each cell contains the full complement of genes for its organism, but only activates a small subset. Hence there are many genes that may never be expressed, or expressed only in some cells, or under some circumstances. Genes provide an inheritance of possible proteins, but the cell itself dictates which ones to turn on and off moment by moment given the circumstances it finds itself in.[12] Those circumstances are the result of the environment the person chooses – diet, exercise and lifestyle.

Over their years of service there are many ways in which genes can become damaged, such as during the process of coiling and uncoiling chromosomes, or from viruses or free radicals (by-products of oxidation). Faulty genes can result in abnormal proteins, which can damage or cause the death of a cell, or cause a cell to replicate uncontrollably, forming cancers.[13] The cell has many processes that can repair or limit the damage of faulty genes. One reason why antioxidants are so important to health is their protective role in preventing free radical damage to DNA.

Cells and networks in action[14]

If we could see the brain in action, we would see a branching network of blood vessels, with blood pumping through the arteries and rushing along the tiny capillaries to nourish every brain cell. The living brain is also a continual electrical and chemical buzz, each neuron like a tiny point of flashing light in the organised chaos of thought. Brain imaging makes use of this continual activity, using different recording methods to measure which neurons and regions are firing more strongly in response to different mental tasks.

In all this hive of activity, what parts of the brain constitute our thoughts, feelings and memories?

Lights – action – thinking

The brain modulates what we are doing and thinking by sending and receiving electrical impulses and chemical signals between the individual neurons and groups of neurons. Thoughts are encoded by the firing of neurons, which involves generating a small pulse of electricity. Impulses travel along neurons at 100 metres per second (360 kilometres per hour), six times faster than the usual speed limit for driving in the city.

The permanent records of memory are laid down in the patterns of neurons – the way they physically connect to one another, and also the strength of connections between them. Neurons with short axons connect to neighbouring cells and those with longer ones connect to neurons in other regions.

Synapses

The axon of one neuron connects to the dendrites of another at small junctions (gaps) called synapses, which play a role in both the transmissions of thoughts and also the storage of long-term memories. Impulses need to cross from one neuron to another for the smooth flow of thought to occur, but the synapses are uncrossable to signals in electrical form. Synapses are only 20 nanometres across (a nanometre is a millionth part of a metre) but like a light globe with a broken filament, the small electrical impulses produced by the neuron cannot cross the gap, no matter how small. The neurons solve this problem by changing their electrical signals into a chemical form. The sending cell releases a neurotransmitter, one of a large range of chemical molecules, which crosses the synaptic gap and fits into a receptor molecule on the receiving neuron. This process is like handing on the baton in a relay race.

Synapses are the sites of memory and record how quickly and easily two neurons communicate. The process is like building up a river crossing. If each person who successfully crosses a river leaves behind a stone, then over time the crossing would become quicker and easier. To make the changes at a synapse permanent, new proteins are made and the physical structures upgraded. Ultimately, genes are the keys to the proteins that fix memories in the brain. When we recall an event from the past, new proteins are made, which means there are continual slight differences in the memory itself over time.[15]

The surprising thing about neurons is that their electrical impulses are remarkably stereotyped. The overall system is similar to electricity in a home. In the kitchen it can turn on the toaster, in the lounge room it could turn on the TV. Electricity is the same no matter where it is in the home. Similarly, the neuron's impulse is important only because of the patterns of connections that the neuron makes with other neurons and with parts of the body. Connect the neuron to a muscle in the arm, and the arm will receive the signal. If the same neuron were rewired to connect to the foot, the foot would receive the signal.[16]

Neurotransmitters[17]

We have described neurotransmitters as chemical molecules whose job is to carry electrical impulses across the synaptic gap. They also diffuse widely throughout the brain carrying signals to receptors in many different regions. Numerous synaptic arrangements, as well as the classic one described above, are known, involving signals that can be propagated in either direction or make use of diffuse distribution of neurotransmitters.

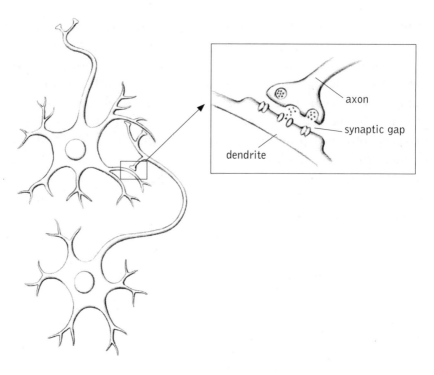

Two neurons showing the axon of one contacting the dendrites of another.
The inset shows how the neurotransmitters cross the synaptic gap.

At least 80 neurotransmitters have been identified which deal with the travelling messages in very different ways.[18] For example:

- Acetylcholine plays a key role in sleep, wakefulness and arousal, and is important for attention, learning and memory.[19] Deficiencies cause memory problems.

- Serotonin is known as the 'feel-good' chemical. It affects mood, with high levels being associated with serenity and optimism. It is linked to many different mental processes with multiple pathways through the brain, including pain, appetite, sleep and blood pressure.[20]

- Glutamate is the brain's main excitatory neurotransmitter. It plays a role in long-term memory, and also possibly in recruiting neurons into large-scale assemblies.[21]

- Dopamine controls arousal levels, and is involved in physical movement, emotion and attention. When it is low, a person cannot make voluntary physical movements and when it is high they feel euphoric.[22]

- Noradrenalin raises physical and mental arousal levels, and is activated by stress. It increases heart rate and blood pressure and decreases intestinal activity, preparing for immediate action.[23] When the stress passes, acetylcholine is released instead.

As is clear from these few examples, none of the neurotransmitters is restricted to a single function. Rather, each one participates in a range of functions, and any one function, such as sleep, depends on a range of neurotransmitters. Each neurotransmitter is secreted by a different type of cell, however, each one has several different sub-types of receptors that allow it to make very specific connections throughout the brain.[24]

Malfunctions occur if there is too little or too much neurotransmitter. For example, too little dopamine is associated with Parkinson's disease and too much with schizophrenia.[25] Low levels of acetylcholine are characteristic of Alzheimer's disease.

Addictive drugs such as LSD and morphine have a similar structure to the transmitters. They attach to the post-synaptic receptor sites and interfere with the normal neurotransmitters.

Networks[26]

By the time we are adults our mental landscapes are so individual that no two of us will see anything in quite the same way. [27]

We have seen in previous sections that neurons are the basic machinery of thinking and memories are ultimately stored as proteins in the synapses between neurons. However, an individual synapse or even a cell doesn't have meaning by itself, just as a single point of colour on a TV or computer screen doesn't have meaning. It is the patterns on a TV screen that make up the pictures we understand. Similarly, it is the patterns of neurons that make up a thought. When we have a different thought, a different set of neurons is firing. The continual fluidity of the brain means that the same patterns are never exactly reproduced.

Neurons with similar function are grouped together in columns that extend through the 2 millimetre thickness of the cortex.[28] One neuron on its own has virtually no impact and would not even blink an eyelid![29] To make an impact, a neuron must fire in concert with hundreds of its fellows. 'Each of the 100 billion nerve cells can be connected in this way to as many as 100,000 other nerve cells. Unimaginable complexity!'[30]

Neurons link up into vast networks of interconnected cells. These networks have intricate connections, like a telephone system that may look haphazard but actually has a clear function underlying its links. Neurons can link to other neurons within the same region, or across widely different regions.

> *I have heard that using your mind, e.g. reading, discussing, listening, can actually help to create new pathways in the brain – is this so? I'd like more about this.*
> EDNA

New neural connections are made with every incoming scrap of information and the brain reacts to this, so old patterns are modified into newer patterns. The process is like a continuing, restless, multi-faceted conversation between various regions of the brain. It is these connections that increase when something new is learned, or old memories reinforced.

The formation of neurons in the brain is mostly completed before birth. There are vastly more neurons than are needed, and those neurons that do not actively begin the process of networking are elbowed out by energetically growing ones.

In early childhood there is vigorous growth of the branches and connections and interconnections, partly dictated by the genetic code of each cell, but guided also by the individual experiences of each child. Networks continue to grow throughout our lives.

Different regions for different memories

Where in our brains are our memories stored? We know that ultimately the synapses between neurons record the events of our lives, but which neurons? Are they all the same, and can anything be stored anywhere?

It turns out that the brain has many regions, each with specialised roles, but all contribute seemlessly to how we perceive and remember events, knowledge and skills.[31]

> *No single memory region exists, and many parts of the brain participate in the representation of any single event … The modern view is that memory is widely distributed but that different areas store different aspects of the whole. There is little redundancy or reduplication of function across these areas. Specific brain regions have specialised functions, and … each contributes in a different way to the storage of whole memories.*[32]

Exactly what is the balance of specialisation and connectedness is gradually being revealed but it is useful to think of the brain as an orchestra and memory as a symphony.[33] No one instrument, or even several like instruments, could play a symphony alone. Each type of musical instrument has a part to play and together they make an integrated whole.

Left and right hemispheres

Just as the body is almost symmetrical, so also the two hemispheres of the brain are almost mirror images of each other. The right side of the brain controls the left side of the body and the left side controls the right side of the body. The hemispheres are joined by a thick swathe of nerve fibres called the corpus callosum, running across the middle the brain. A person cannot function competently if either side suffers major damage (unless the damage occurred in early childhood when there is still flexibility in the arrangements of the neural networks).

The hemispheres have subtle differences in their higher mental functions, in particular with the left side specialised for language and the right side for spatial processing. In left-handed people the lateralisation is often symmetrically reversed, but not always. Current thinking is that the brain was originally almost completely symmetrical, and that tool use and language were primary forces in the lateralisation of the hominid brain.

Each hemisphere seems to have a characteristic way of processing information, with the left side of the brain more analytic and the right side more holistic. Interestingly, the lateralisation for language also shows in how music is appreciated. Brain images of musicians were recorded over years of training. Initially, the non-trained music lovers listened more holistically, involving sensory perceptions and emotions, and the right hemisphere was most active. As the years and their training progressed, the analytic left brain areas became more dominant when they listened to music.[34] Sign language is similarly intriguing, activating the language areas of the left hemisphere in the same way as speech does, even though the original words in Sign are visuo-spatial rather than auditory.

Some writers refer to the hemispheres as having rivalry and others use the word cooperation. They are rivals in the sense that one or the other takes charge in any given situation. Otherwise there could be confusion, which is thought to happen in stuttering. It is useful to think of the two halves as having favourite jobs to do as well as keeping each other informed about what is going on. Both sides are used in cooperative tasks such as using tools and other physical activities.[35]

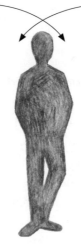

LEFT HEMISPHERE

controls right side of body, and also analytic thinking and symbolic processes like:

- language and the hand signs of formal Sign
- logic
- numbers
- sequence
- reading
- writing

RIGHT HEMISPHERE

controls left side of body, and also holistic thinking like:

- visualisation and coding pictures
- imagination
- colour
- spatial skills and hand gestures
- melody and rhythm of music
- environmental noises
- autobiographical memory
- whole face recognition

Each hemisphere of the brain has specialised jobs to do, as well as sharing information with the other side.

In general, the two hemispheres have different ways of thinking, with the left hemisphere forming plans and pursuing them, and tending to ignore or deny discrepancies that don't fit the overall ideas. The right side looks for discrepancies, and is more like a devil's advocate. Dominance between these two types of thinking alternates over a period of hours.[36]

There is a simple method that dates back to ancient times to find out which hemisphere is currently dominant. Breathing is controlled alternately by left and right sides and usually one side is dominant. To determine which one is more active, cover each nostril in turn and see which side breathes more freely. If the brain is over-busy at night before sleeping, the right nostril is usually more open, indicating the detail-oriented, left hemisphere is in control. Some advocates of left brain/right brain differentiation such as Angela Booth attribute even more differences to left and right sides:

> *If I'm in left brain mode, I won't feel like writing. I'll want to procrastinate and read a magazine or check my e-mail. If I want to get writing straight away, I'll put my finger against my right nostril for ten breaths, which changes my breathing to left nostril dominance, and hence my right brain dominance.*[37]

The four lobes of the brain[38]

Each hemisphere of the brain is divided into four lobes, which have specific roles to play in memory as well as general thinking. The cortex is the outer layer of each lobe and is shaped into patterns of bumps and folds (called gyri and sulci) which are the same among most people, although no two brains are exactly alike.

- The visual lobes are located at the back of the brain. They comprise 70 per cent of the sensory regions of the brain, and each one has over 30 different sub-regions that are used to understand the visual world in terms of movement, colour and shape.

- The parietal lobes are located in front of the visual lobes. They are concerned with touch, pain, temperature and proprioception (where you are in space), and each lobe has a special region called the somatosensory cortex that is laid out as a complete map of the body's sensors. During brain surgery, if the neurons at any spot on the somatosensory cortex are electrically stimulated, the person feels that the corresponding part of the body has been touched.

- The temporal lobes are located beneath the parietal lobes. The temporal cortices process auditory information (pitch and rhythm) deciding if it is speech, music or noise, and the left temporal cortex helps translate words into thoughts. Deep within each temporal lobe is the hippocampus and related structures important for episodic memories.

- The frontal lobes are located at the front third of the brain, with a major fissure dividing them from the parietal lobes. They are involved in taking action to make things happen, including planning, judgement, decision making and motor control. Both left and right frontal lobes have a motor cortex that is laid out as a body map similar to the somatosensory region, except that it drives our muscles rather than listening to our sensors. If neurons at a spot on this map are electrically stimulated, the corresponding muscle in the body contracts. At the very front of the brain are the prefrontal cortices, which are involved in maintaining concentration during working memory tasks through feedback loops with other regions of the brain. The prefrontal cortices also seem to be important for creating a personal perspective on things through continual exchanges of viewpoint with the limbic system.[39]

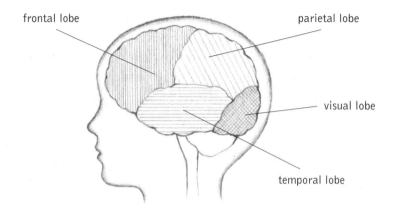

The left side of the brain showing the four lobes.
The right side is a mirror image of it.

Studies have shown that the parts of the brain that we use more often recruit additional neurons and increase in size. In one study volunteers did a sequence of finger movements and after prolonged training, they could perform the sequence at twice the speed. Of particular interest, the area in the motor cortex that was activated by the task increased in size and stayed larger for several weeks.[40] Similarly, studies of taxi drivers in London have shown an increase in the areas that are thought to encode spatial maps, with larger regions for those who had been driving the longest.[41] These studies show that when we practise a skill, the brain literally donates more power to the task.

When brain imaging is used to find which areas 'light up' when certain mental tasks are done, the tests often show a main area and perhaps several other active areas. Information can be distributed across several different regions.

Semantic memory

Semantic memories seem to follow the general principle that the part of the brain that is most used in learning some information is the likely place where its long-term memories are stored. Thus, knowledge of things we learn about through their visual appearance, such as animals and plants, are stored in the visual association areas, whereas things we learn about through our actions, such as tools, are remembered in the association areas of the motor cortex in the frontal lobe.[42]

How the brain remembers words is interesting, because we both hear and speak them. Two regions in the left hemisphere are particularly involved in processing words; one in the auditory region called Wernicke's area – involved in the meanings of words – and one in the frontal cortex called Broca's area – involved with the grammar of words. People who can speak fluently but have trouble understanding spoken words are likely to have a problem with Wernicke's area. Conversely, when we know exactly what we want to say but cannot make grammatical sentences to express ourselves, the problem is likely to be in Broca's area.

The central problem for the Memory Survey respondents was forgetting names. What we have seen is that all the lobes of the brain are involved in storing semantic knowledge (which includes names of people and everything we know about them). The diversity of regions helps to explain why we can see a person and know exactly who they are, and yet be unable to retrieve the sounds of their name. The name is stored in a different area from their other information and is not activated sufficiently strongly. It also helps to explain why the name might suddenly pop up when we remember many different things about the person. The regions are interconnected, and activity in one region can stimulate related knowledge in another.

As we age there are minor losses of neurons in different regions, which are unique to each person. Problems of juggling many tasks at once may be due to the synchronisation needed to get all areas talking to each other. At one time or another we have all felt slightly out of sync with ourselves, perhaps clumsy or slower than usual. These are probably synchronisation glitches, and as we become more alert the brain gets in step with itself (such as with the first cup of tea or coffee for the day or as we move around and get the blood circulating).

Episodic memory

Episodic memories differ from semantic ones because they describe specific events, so information about sights and sounds and touch need to be associated with the time and place they occurred.

The hippocampus, frontal cortex and amygdala all play a part in making the component parts of an episodic memory into a coherent whole. Much is still to be learned about the intricate details of this process, but it is likely that specific feedback circuits are involved. To be conscious of an action, the temporal lobes need to be active. From imaging studies we know that when an episode is encoded, the left frontal cortex is more active, but when we remember the event later, the right frontal cortex becomes active.[43]

When we have trouble remembering who told us something interesting, the problem is probably due to the frontal cortex not being able to recall the appropriate context for the information, such as when or where we heard it. Fragments of memory can often be disconnected from their original sources and reconnected to some other similar event, or merged with other events that might have occurred.

The right prefrontal cortex is also necessary for maintaining attention and goal-directed action, particularly in the face of distractions. Simple lapses of attention, such as losing your train of thought, are thought to be due to a slow wave of electrical activity that passes over the frontal region. The slow wave lasts for a fraction of a second and disrupts the attentional circuit. It is a common occurrence, increasing in frequency with age, and appears to be due to fluctuations in the neural networks that underlie attention.[44]

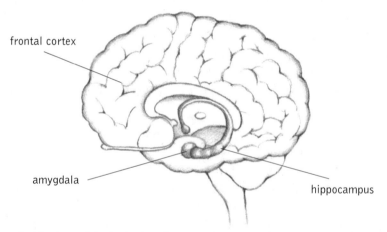

A side view of the brain showing areas important for episodic memory.

Emotional content of memories

Events also carry with them their emotional significance. The amygdala has been much studied for its role in memory of fearful events and the persistence of unwanted memories. It is composed of many sub-regions that coordinate the body's response to fear, such as increasing heart rate, freezing body movements and slowing digestion. Some of them may be involved in our general levels of anxiety and others in responding to specific cues that cause an immediate flight or fight response.[45] The amygdala has an interactive relationship with the release of hormones such as adrenaline and cortisol.[46]

We can startle easily to a loud noise, then quickly realise that it is not a threat, because information about events travels to the amygdala along two pathways.[47] One pathway provides a relatively direct route from the sensors, taking about 12 milliseconds. The other route travels through the cortex, which can make more informed decisions about the event, but takes half as long again.

Implicit memory

Implicit memory occurs in all regions of the brain. The priming part of implicit memory can be thought of as 'warming up' the sensory systems in specific areas: visual priming in primary and secondary visual areas, sounds in auditory areas and touch in somatosensory areas. When the neural network of a region has been recently active it retains a little of that activity, which makes it faster to respond later. Words that we have heard recently will be recognised or named quicker than those that have not been mentioned for some time.

Other aspects of implicit memory draw on specific regions. When learning a new physical skill such as typing (or dancing, or golf) for the first time, the cerebellum (the 'little brain' beneath the visual lobe) is important for the coordination and timing of skilled movements.[48] The cerebellum is also involved in non-conscious linking of stimuli to rewards.

Concepts

> We humans are geniuses at distillation – we automatically take the
> buzzing, teeming richness of experience and find a manageable set
> of objects or laws.[49]

Categories of things we see or hear or touch are formed by the gradual building up of knowledge about what certain items have in common. Finding the essential similarity between several items can happen without our conscious awareness, and seems to take place in the original regions where the information is first processed – the visual, auditory and somatosensory association areas.[50] We can also intentionally group items into categories and we do this all the time – food, household items, clothes, even people, which involves the temporal lobe, in particular the hippocampal system.[51] Exactly how categories are stored has many different tentative explanations, but one that is consistent with the other information we know about memory is that they are represented in terms of the relationships we have with them, rather than their physical appearance.[52]

Current research into brain regeneration

It was initially assumed that no new brain cells could be formed after birth. Recently, however, researchers have found evidence that this is not the case. We describe below how new cells are formed in the brain.

Cell birth (neurogenesis)[53]

Every human begins as a single cell. The cell divides, and then its daughter cells divide, again and again, growing and maturing into the baby, then the child and then the adult. The very first cells in the embryo are stem cells, which are the precursors to all other cells. They have simple shapes and perform no specialised functions. As the embryo develops, most of the cells specialise into different kinds, some into muscle, others skin or brain. These cells migrate to appropriate sites and then link up with surrounding cells to form the complex structures of the body organs, skin, muscle and brain, differentiating further in the process.

The process by which stem cells in the brain divide and differentiate to form neurons is called neurogenesis. Brain cells develop in a series of stages. First, they start as general purpose stem cells, able to differentiate into any kind of cell in the brain or body. When they divide, some become committed as precursors to the specialised cells of the brain (including neurons and glial cells). These committed stem cells can then divide again and the progeny that are destined to make neurons are called neuroblasts. Finally, neuroblasts migrate to appropriate locations, such as the output region of the hippocampus where they differentiate into neurons, with their characteristic shapes and functions.

Previously, studies of a variety of animals (from canaries and rats to humans) have shown that stem cells – the precursors to neurons – are found in many parts of the brain. Most of these cells don't appear to develop further and it was assumed that the brain could not repair itself using such stem cells. However, evidence has been gradually accumulating that in many animals there are selected regions – among them the hippocampus (important for forming new memories) – in which stem cells do continue to develop into functioning brain cells.[54]

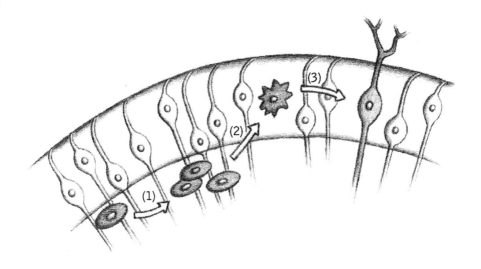

(1) The formation of new neurons begins with stem cells which divide;
(2) the daughter cells migrate to appropriate locations in the hippocampus; and
(3) finally differentiate into neurons.[55]

A critical question for humans is whether new brain cells are made in sufficient numbers to be useful, and what factors affect their use in maintaining and repairing brain function both in normal ageing and in treating brain diseases. Not surprisingly, understanding such factors is a hot topic of research. A clear picture of how neurogenesis is controlled is yet to emerge, but there are some promising leads.

The first evidence that neurogenesis was even possible in humans was not collected until the late 1990s. This groundbreaking discovery was of natural, spontaneous cell birth, occurring without interference from the medical team. It was only possible to know what had happened because of the tracing of new cells. Five patients who suffered from cancer of the tongue or larynx were being given a benign substance that could help trace the dividing cells of tumours. The substance also marked other dividing cells, and hence could show where new cells were being made. The marker was found in a kind of neuron called a granule cell, in a region of the hippocampus called the dentate gyrus. The discovery provided the first proof of adult human neurogenesis.

Why, if the brain has the ability to create new neurons, does it seem so reluctant to do so? After all, there are stem cells in many different brain regions, but they don't appear to divide or specialise to create new neurons.

There may be good reasons for the brain's reluctance to create new neurons all the time. The brain is a complex organ, and its smooth functioning is necessary for ongoing survival. Adding new neurons is like rewiring a computer that controls a Boeing 747. Any tinkering with the controls should happen while the jet is not in the middle of a critical manoeuvre! Preferably not during flight at all.

Ongoing research has shown that neurogenesis seems to be inhibited by a variety of factors, including certain everyday inputs, and some excitatory neurotransmitters and hormones that are released by stress.

Factors that affect neurogenesis[56]

Neurogenesis is known to be enhanced by enriched environments, as was discovered with studies on mice. Both physical exercise and new learning tasks seem to play important but different roles. In one study, comparing environments with and without running wheels, mice with running wheels ended up with twice as many new neurons as their sedentary counterparts. Running seems to promote stem cell division whereas new learning tasks seem to promote survival and differentiation of the stem cell progeny. Importantly, old mice benefited from enriched environments just as young ones did, although with much lower levels of neurogenesis than younger mice.

There is, no doubt, much more to be discovered, and these results are yet to be demonstrated in humans. However, they are consistent with advice that aerobic exercise has a major effect in maintaining good memory, and keeping mentally active is also beneficial. Lowering stress levels may also play an important role in promoting the stages that lead to new neurons.

In other approaches, the molecular compounds underlying neurogenesis are being explored. One substance, when injected into rats, produced marked proliferation of stem cells and another promoted production of neurons. A future step will be to show whether such cells can be effectively integrated into normal brain function in humans.

Other current studies involve comparing the genes active in brain regions that display neurogenesis with the patterns of those in regions that don't. If the genes could be identified, the proteins they produce would be an important piece in solving the puzzle of neurogenesis.

Therapeutic approaches may eventually involve multiple levels of intervention, including changes to physical and mental environments, supplying key regulatory molecules, using gene therapy, and stem cell transplants. The eventual goal is to be able to trace the long chain of events that leads through all stages of neurogenesis, and be able to induce neuronal regeneration as required.

At a glance

Many levels of knowledge contribute to our understanding
of memory in the brain:

- Our memories are a unique combination of biological
  inheritance plus an individual's lifetime experiences. Our genes
  dictate that our brains are human ones, but our synapses are
  our own.[57]

- Genes determine which proteins can be made, but whether they
  are activated or not depends on the environment.

- Synapses are the sites of memory storage, where new proteins
  are made to form long-term memories.

- Neurotransmitters are the chemical messengers of the brain
  and are important for the formation of memories, as well as
  other body aspects such as mood, arousal and sleep.

- Neurons are the hi-tech processors of the brain, and their
  electrical and chemical signals are the basis of all thought.
  They continue to branch and form networks throughout life.

- Many regions of the brain contribute to the memory of an
  event, with memories from different senses (vision, hearing and
  touch) being processed in different regions and brought together
  in the hippocampus.

- Recent research has shown that neurogenesis is possible
  and may indeed be normal in some brain regions, although
  more needs to be learned before therapeutic applications are
  practicable.

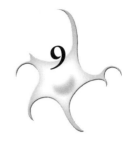

9

Lifelong Memory
Lifelong Learning

Memory is the glue that binds our mental life,
the scaffolding that holds our personal history
and that makes it possible to grow and change
throughout life.[1]

We set out to write a book about memory for everyday living and we found that the ability to remember was not a stand-alone entity. We also had to write about the brain system – the encoding, storage and retrieval of memories – and the geography of the brain that handles, supports and enables the three phases of memory. Memory is not one single thing, but rather a collection of expert systems fine-tuned to record for the future the things that we do, the facts that we know and skills that we know how to do. The system must also forget the mass of unwanted trivia, an important built-in ability of the brain. Sometimes needed information goes too, so strategies to take charge of our memories was central to our book plan.

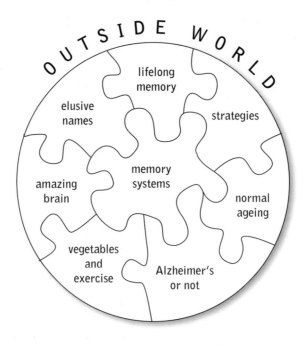

Memory is part of many interlocking aspects of life.

Because we wanted, above all, for the book to bring understanding, comfort and usefulness to people's lives, we needed to include what happens to memory with ageing and the differences between normal forgetfulness and dementia diseases. We also outlined the first steps for doing something about early memory loss.

Memory and thinking are highly valued yet surprisingly easy to nourish by the quite ordinary and abundant things of life, such as oxygen through the blood supply and vitamins and antioxidants from vegetables and fruit. 'Memory' need not just happen to people, but rather can be maintained and improved with a basic understanding of how the memory system works within the intricacies of the brain.

One survey respondent asked of memory, 'Is it true that you use it or lose it?' 'Yes!' is the emphatic answer given by the scientific literature as well as the everyday wisdom of ordinary people. Staying involved, keeping up social contacts, relearning forgotten but important names – with a strategy to keep them in place – are all part of a recipe to keep and enjoy a healthy memory.

In Chapters 1 to 8 we have relayed the distilled knowledge of the experts. These chapters are like maps, describing current knowledge. Some help us directly manage our memories, like the strategies described in Chapters 3 and 4, and some apply indirectly, such as the health issues raised in Chapter 7. Like the interlocking pieces of a jigsaw puzzle, the chapters show different aspects of how we understand memory. All are interconnected.

If a map shows us the extent of the territory, a compass gives us a direction. The map of mind and body systems we share with all mankind, but the direction each person should go is individual. To make good decisions one needs across-the-board information. The aim of this book has been to provide readers with the understanding they need for self-help for memory problems, which was a prevailing theme in the Memory Survey responses. For a full appreciation of the memory systems, we must firmly anchor memory in the brain, the amazing body organ that is both physical and mental.

Incomparable memory

The great power of the human brain is not in storing facts but in having ideas.[2]

The Memory Surveys revealed a deep interest in how remembering works. We emphasise that memory is so much more than just a record of our experiences. Memory can be compared variously to a library, a powerhouse and a computer. Each can serve to illustrate a point, but none quite captures the fascinating complexity of the human memory system. If it's a library, it's one where the books read each other and powerful information leaks out.[3] If it's a powerhouse, it's one that self-services and does not need a lot of space. If it's a computer, it's one that generates its own ideas, making meaning out of its world.

For centuries people have stored some of their memories outside their minds, inscribing them with brush or ink. Whenever a culture has had an external way of storing information, the technology of that time and place has also been used as a metaphor for memory, and a way to understand the extent of its capabilities.

Does anyone remember microfiche? It was a system of putting large amounts of information on small plastic sheets that could be read by a special machine. Microfiche began to replace the library system of one index card per book. H.G. Wells, writing in 1937, welcomed the arrival of the invention with expansive enthusiasm:

There is no practical obstacle whatever now to the creation of an efficient index to all human knowledge, ideas and achievements, to the creation, that is, of a complete planetary memory for all mankind ... The whole human memory can be, and probably in a short time will be, made accessible to every individual.[4]

As a metaphor for memory, microfiche missed a vital feature. Memory is more than a complete record of information. Ideas link with each other. One idea connects and calls up the next, which links to others to make networks.

As a memory device, microfiche was rapidly superseded by computers, although few people envisaged just how successful they would be. Few people – even with such creative, imaginative minds as H.G. Wells – could have predicted their rise and widespread use. In the mid-20th century, Thomas Watson, chairman of IBM, is reported to have said, 'I think there is a world market for maybe five computers.'[5] At the start of the 21st century, a newspaper reported that the billionth computer had been sold.[6] Computers have become so absorbed into our lifestyles that many of them go unnoticed. Even if we don't use a computer with a monitor and keyboard, they are present in such commonplace things as washing machines and cars.

Amazing though the advent of computers was, an even bigger surprise of the late 20th century was communication systems. A revolution in the mass storage of information and its distribution emerged in the 1990s with the advent of the World Wide Web. Consider the task of looking for information on vitamin supplements. Our starting point is a popular search engine, which has dozens of links to pages on the topic. We skim through them quickly, finding what we seek at a university research centre that specialises in food nutrition. We also see (and try to ignore) countless ads and other distractions.

As the most recent technological metaphor for memory, the web has some interesting similarities. Ideas in memory are useful in their own right, but also call up other ideas, just as pages on the web do. They both have seemingly unlimited capacity – the limits of human memory are restricted only by motivation and attention, and the web is estimated at well over a billion pages and still growing.[7] Both memory and the web also allow very rapid access to their information starting from a key phrase or idea.

Memory and the web also have many foibles in common. Both are full of junk, search engines are not perfect, and even when one knows that information exists one cannot always find the right links to reach it. Information is being created and removed all the time, with gems of knowledge interspersed with useless stuff and a multitude of distractions.

Ultimately, of course, memory is a multi-faceted thing that is truly only like itself. Memory and cognition are natural properties of a brain that is by nature curious and eager for stimulation, one that doesn't just record experiences but makes sense out of them.

The mind is the brain in action

We have discussed how technology can be used to store large amounts of public knowledge and how those devices can be compared to memory. We now turn to the 'I' feeling in the mind that seems like the essential self.

The elusive part of being human lies in the mental realm – having awareness of self and knowing that others have awareness of themselves, using language and knowing that others understand us. The physical body – the skin, tissues, blood, organs and bones – seems easier to understand. Superficially, it seems that there are two of us, a physical self and the 'I' self.

Because that 'I' seems only partly in charge of what goes on within ourselves it's easy to have a sense of duality. Back in 1637, the philosopher René Descartes thought that mind represented all that was lofty in human nature and the body was in some way just for the baser things of life. In fact the duality is an illusion. Current brain science recognises that mind and body are two parts of one system.

The relationship between mind and body is a close one. They grew up together, so to speak. The explanation of 'Descartes' error' is argued eloquently and scientifically by Antonio Damasio in his book of that name.[8] There is a different duality that Damasio does support, that of the reason and the emotions. Objective reasoning takes place in the frontal cortex, but evaluation of whether something should be done or not done is the province of the emotional centre in the limbic system. If the reasoning part of the brain makes a 'map' of the pros and cons of a given situation, the limbic system supplies the 'compass' that decides which actions are worth taking. The neuroscience view of emotion is that it is far more necessary for balanced living than the everyday dismissive view that emotions are inferior to reasoning.

The popular saying 'minds are what brains do' encapsulates the idea that mind and body are inseparable. An analogy with a car is that driving is what cars do. Not all the time, of course, since they need servicing, and are often parked for long periods of time, but intrinsically, driving is the reason for cars, their most characteristic behaviour. Minds are not 'in' the brain, in the same sense that driving is not 'in' a car. The mind is the brain in action, two views of the same system.

The conscious and non-conscious partnership

The brain (and through it the mind) works with information it receives from the eyes, ears and other senses, from stored memories and from the messages about the ongoing state of the body organs, muscles and systems. Such messages might be about the need for food and water. The body and brain are regulated by a complex interplay of biochemistry and firing of neurons. The compilation of all this information is a huge business. There are far too many bits of information to hold in working memory, evaluate and respond appropriately in the single stream of consciousness that we think of as the self. The conscious self couldn't deal with so much information so quickly. So it doesn't. A huge amount of brain activity goes on below our level of awareness.

Our sense of self is constructed through all our memories of who we are and where we have been, and is assembled from both conscious and non-conscious parts. We are conscious of our own general knowledge and the events of our lives. We are conscious of our own stream of consciousness – second by second – perceiving, deliberating and making decisions. In parallel with the conscious self, the many parts of the non-conscious self are also processing information – millisecond by millisecond – accessing our non-conscious memories and only drawing them to our attention when the circumstances warrant it. The conscious and non-conscious minds form an intricate cooperative system that is still being unravelled. The feeling that we are not always fully in control of our minds is a legitimate one – the non-conscious mind does not need our conscious control. It is an equal partner with our conscious self and together with it, works for our benefit.

Memory for life

In a complex world of constant change, where knowledge becomes obsolete every few years, education can no longer be something that one acquires during youth to serve for an entire lifetime. Rather education must focus on instilling the ability to continue learning throughout life.[9]

'Learn something new every day' is an old adage that still holds good. The skills we need for a changing world are 'how to find out' rather than trying to know everything. No one learns all the technology of their own time, let alone that of the future. Within living memory the world has seen several technological revolutions, as calculators replaced slide rules and computers replaced calculators. But constant change is not just an illusion, technology has allowed faster processing of all sorts of things, from digital cameras to images on the TV screen.[10]

When we know how to find out, we don't have to do everything ourselves. Flexibility means coming to terms with change, and memory is the tool we use to do so. It's about knowing which school child to ask to program the video, find information on the web or set up an email account. Artist Jeanette Harper emphasises flexibility in her recipe for a changing world. 'To survive and grow, get a healthy life style, be flexible and open minded, when necessary embrace change, retain flexibility of mind and body, play a part in the life of the community, be part of many worlds.'[11]

The daughters of memory

As we come to the end of our time with you it is fitting to draw back from the details of the previous chapters and see memory across time and space. Memory has fascinated philosophers, writers and scientists, as well as featuring in mythologies, since time immemorial. It gives the ability to pan out and see other times and places with the perspective of distance. Rather than just the stories of our own lives, it gives those of people everywhere and every-when.

We sit, looking out the window. We see a lofty mountain peak, home of the gods of ancient Greece including Mnemosyne, goddess of memory. Her daughters, the three Muses, embodied the gracious things of life, music, poetry, drama, judgement and wisdom.[12] The idea that memory is the mother of judgement and wisdom is very much relevant to our time. Wisdom comes from the long accumulation of facts and knowledge, experiences, actions, and common sense, and gives insights into deciding the best choice in any given situation.

Flexible thinking is needed to look at old knowledge in a new way, making use of the discoveries of others. Recent findings about the role of antioxidants in protecting brain cells brings an added sweetness to the taste of fresh vegetables. Food science has unravelled a huge amount of detail about how the body uses the food we give it and what it does with the excess fat. New scanning technology can now illuminate (in technicolour) what brain cells are doing when we think and remember. Our gratitude goes out to the virtual army of volunteers who walked so that studies could measure how much we need to puff to improve the oxygen levels in the blood flow to brain capillaries.

What is new in memory research is not so much what we need to do to improve memory, but the reasons why it works. We think of this book as being both a map and a compass. If the map is all the information, the compass is pointing back to the brain for literally everything we do. Memory is just one part of a fantastic, interconnected system that both affects memory and is monitored and recorded by it. Like all good friendships, it responds well to care and attention and in return has our best interests at heart.

U3A

The University of the Third Age (U3A) is a unique, non-profit organisation that promotes lifelong learning. There are no examinations and no entrance standard is required. There are courses in literature, language, astronomy, politics, ecology – in fact almost anything where a leader will volunteer their expertise. Discussion groups set their own topics and ways of conducting their meetings. What a way to set the brain cells buzzing! One does not of course need to join a group to find mental stimulation, but the presence and contribution of others brings an extra dimension, a mental stretching of one's thinking that can be very exciting.

Further Reading

For updates on the information in this book, see *The Memory Book* website
www.thememorybook.org

Carter, Rita, *Mapping the Mind*, Phoenix, London, 2000. With clear language and
good illustrations, Carter covers a vast range of topics in this fascinating tour
of brain country. She makes accessible the latest knowledge of all aspects of the
workings of the brain.

Damasio, Antonio R., *Descartes' Error: Emotion, Reason and the Human Brain*,
Avon Books, New York, 1994. With good science and persuasive language, Damasio
dispels the myth that the rational region of the brain is somehow on a higher plain
than the emotional. He shows how their interaction is essential for good decision
making and balanced living.

Greenfield, Susan, *Brain Story: Unlocking Our Inner World of Emotions, Memories,
Ideas and Desires*, BBC Worldwide, London, 2000. With a light touch and beautiful
pictures, and based on her BBC TV series, this book is a pleasant and interesting
introduction to the mind and memory.

Pinel, John P. J., *Biopsychology*, 3rd edition, Allyn & Bacon, Needham Heights, MA,
1997. A high-quality resource book with a wealth of technical detail about memory
and the brain. Attractive illustrations enhance every page and add clarity to
in-depth explanations.

Savige, Gayle; Wahlqvist, Mark; Lee, Daniel and Snelson, Brett, *ageFIT: Fitness and
nutrition for an independent future*, Pan Macmillan, Sydney, 2001. A team of experts
have contributed a fund of knowledge in a very readable book about fitness and
nutrition. They clearly describe the role that a healthy lifestyle plays in supporting
overall good health and creating the physical basis of a good memory, and provide
pages of practical guidance such as checklists of food groups.

Schacter, Daniel L., *The Seven Sins of Memory*, Houghton Mifflin, New York, 2001.
Schacter has selected seven major areas where our memories can fail us and deals
with each failing with entertaining anecdotes as well as first-rate science. He explains
the counter-intuitive idea that each one can also be viewed as a blessing in disguise.

Squire, Larry R. and Kandel, Eric, R., *Memory: From Mind to Molecules*, Scientific
American Library. Distributed by W. H. Freeman and Company, New York, 1999.
A psychologist and a biologist have combined to write an excellent and easy-to-
understand book, rich in detail about memory mechanisms and how they are
encoded, stored, recalled, enhanced or diminished. They provide all the technical
details that we really wanted to know about the workings of memory.

Endnotes

Chapter 1
Why Do We Forget Names?

1 Wiles, J. and Wiles, J. (1999). 'Survey on Memory – Summary of Responses', Sydney (unpublished report). A questionnaire was mailed to members of the University of the Third Age (U3A), Sydney, Northern Region in 1998. The Memory Survey included the six questions below, plus an invitation to provide additional comments and anecdotes, a request for the respondent's age bracket and permission to quote from the responses:

1. Have you noticed any memory lapses in yourself?
2. What things do you forget?
3. If you remember later, what prompts the remembering?
4. Which memory lapses worry you most?
5. What tips or strategies or memory aids do you find useful?
6. What memory issues would you like to know more about?

Responses were received from November 1998 to February 1999 from 275 people. All respondents were members of U3A and hence over 50 years of age with the vast majority being over 60. The original results were reported in the U3A Newsletter in 1999 and a summary of responses was mailed to all participants. Quotes from the Memory Survey used in this book are in the respondents' own words, though their names have been changed to protect their privacy.

2 Many respondents reported more than one lapse therefore the percentages add up to more than 100 per cent.

3 Sachs, O. (1991). *Seeing Voices*, Picador, London, p. 49.

4 Schacter, D.L. (2001). *The Seven Sins of Memory*, Houghton Mifflin, New York.

Chapter 2
The Memory System

1 Hampl, P. (1996). 'Memory and Imagination', in McConkey, J. (Ed.), *The Anatomy of Memory: An Anthology*, Oxford University Press, Oxford, p. 211.

2 Squire, L.R. and Kandel, E.R. (1999). *Memory: From Mind to Molecules*, Scientific American Library, New York.

3 For a detailed description see Squire, L.R. and Kandel, E.R. (1999). *Memory: From Mind to Molecules*.

4 Paraphrased from Schacter, D.L. (1996). *Searching for Memory: The Brain, the Mind, and the Past*, Basic Books, New York.

5 Baddeley, A. (1996). *Your Memory: A User's Guide*, Prion, London.

6 Schacter, D.L. (1996). *Searching for Memory: The Brain, the Mind, and the Past*.

7 Squire, L.R. and Kandel, E.R. (1999). *Memory: From Mind to Molecules*.

8 Schacter, D.L. and Buckner, R.L. (1998). 'Priming and the Brain', *Neuron*, Vol. 20, pp. 185–95.

9 Baddeley, A. (1996). *Your Memory: A User's Guide*.

10 Schacter, D.L. (1996). *Searching for Memory: The Brain, the Mind, and the Past*.

11 Squire, L.R. and Kandel, E.R. (1999). *Memory: From Mind to Molecules*.

12 Robbins, A. (1991). *Awaken the Giant Within*, Simon and Schuster, New York.

13 Kandel, E.R. and Hawkins, R. D. (1993). 'The Biological Basis of Learning and Individuality', in *Mind and Brain: Readings from Scientific American*, Scientific American Library, New York, p. 40.

14 Schacter, D.L. (1996). *Searching for Memory: The Brain, the Mind, and the Past*.

15 Schacter, D.L. (1996). *Searching for Memory: The Brain, the Mind, and the Past*.

16 Squire, L.R. and Kandel, E.R. (1999). *Memory: From Mind to Molecules*.

17 Schacter, D.L. (1996). *Searching for Memory: The Brain, the Mind, and the Past*.

18 Schacter, D.L. (2001). *The Seven Sins of Memory*, Houghton Mifflin, New York.

19 In this book we use the familiar term 'recall' to mean bringing information out of memory. The technical term in the memory literature is 'retrieval', which covers recall (using a cue to access memory); recognition (asking a yes/no question); familiarity and spontaneous associations. Many technical books give more detail, for example, see Schacter, D.L. (2001), *The Seven Sins of Memory*, Chapter 2.

20 Interestingly, ghost is almost never the word selected if the question is just 'Name a mythical being', without the rhyme, or just 'Say a word that rhymes with post', without the mythic cue.

21 Schacter, D.L. (2001). *The Seven Sins of Memory*.

22 Proust, M. (1913). 'Swann's Way', in *Remembrance of Things Past*, translated into English by C.K. Scott Moncrief (1922). Reprinted in 1964 Chatto & Windus, London, pp. 60–61.

23 Squire, L.R. and Kandel, E.R. (1999). *Memory: From Mind to Molecules*.

24 Gazzaniga, M.S., Ivry, R.B. and Mangun, G.R. (1998). *Cognitive Neuroscience: The Biology of the Mind*, W.W. Norton & Company, New York, p. 435.

25 Schacter, D.L. (1996). *Searching for Memory: The Brain, the Mind, and the Past*.

Chapter 3
Dealing with Glitches

1 Wiles, J. and Wiles, J. (1999). 'Survey on Memory – Summary of Responses', Sydney (unpublished report).
2 Some advisers advocate ridiculous images, like picturing the face of Barbara with barbed wire wound round it. This idea does not appeal to everyone. Martha (Memory Survey) says 'This is not the way I want to remember friends.' This is understandable, so use the images that appeal to you. We find the barbed-wire image distasteful but in spite of this can't help thinking of it now when we see or hear 'Barbara'. For more names and images, see Pease, A. and Pease, B. (1994). *How to Remember Names, Faces, Lists*, Pease Training International, Avalon Beach, NSW.
3 Schacter, D.L. (2001). *The Seven Sins of Memory*, Houghton Mifflin, New York.
4 Schacter, D.L. (1996). *Searching for Memory: The Brain, the Mind, and the Past*, Basic Books, New York.
5 Schacter, D.L. (2001). *The Seven Sins of Memory*.
6 In a three-day course, people were trained on a system called Photo-fit, designed by Penry and used by the police in identikits. Sets of features taken from real photographs – chins, noses, eyes, types of hair etc. – were put together to construct faces. In subsequent tests, and against all expectations, it was found that the training to recognise faces on such shallow dimensions was no help at all. People who completed the course were the same or worse than others who didn't take the course! In a follow-up study, the memory researchers, Baddeley and Patterson, found that faces encoded on the basis of 'deeper' dimensions such as honesty, liveliness or intelligence are remembered better than those encoded as a set of features. For more details see Baddeley, A. (1996). *Your Memory: A User's Guide*, Prion, London, Chapter 10.
7 Squire, L.R. and Kandel, E.R. (1999). *Memory: From Minds to Molecules*, Scientific American Library, New York.
8 Alan Baddeley calls the part of the brain used for visual mnemonics the visuo-spatial sketchpad. For more details see Baddeley, A. (1996). *Your Memory: A User's Guide*, Chapter 3.
9 Squire, L.R. and Kandel, E.R. (1999). *Memory: From Minds to Molecules*.
10 Lapp, D.C. (1998). *Maximizing Your Memory Power*, 2nd edition, Barron's Educational Series, New York.
11 For more information on T.O.T, a useful reference is Schacter, D.L. (2001). *The Seven Sins of Memory*, Chapter 3.
12 de Bono, E. (1997). *Textbook of Wisdom*, Penguin, London, p. 173.
13 Schacter, D.L. (2001). *The Seven Sins of Memory*.
14 Joyce, James (1994). *Ulysses*, Naxos Audio Books, Germany, CD 4.
15 Baddeley, A. (1996). *Your Memory: A User's Guide*.

Chapter 4
Improving Memory over Time

1   Stine, E.A.L. (1993). 'Commentary: Is Memory Something We Have or Something We Do?', in Davies, G.M. and Logie, R.H. (Eds). *Memory in Everyday Life*, North Holland, Amsterdam, p. 447.
2   Baddeley, A. (1996). *Your Memory: A User's Guide*, Prion, London, pp. 356–63.
3   Buzan, T. (1989). *Use Your Head*, BBC Books, London.
4   Schacter, D.L. (2001). *The Seven Sins of Memory*, Houghton Mifflin, New York.
5   For a very readable account of the relationship between the emotions and the rational mind, see Damasio, A.R. (1994). *Descartes' Error: Emotion, Reason and the Human Brain*, Avon Books, New York.
6   There is much in the scientific literature that deals with traumatic memories but we have found little that takes a scientific approach to dealing with minor annoying memories as a central issue. However, the popular press contains several suggestions which we describe in this section.
7   Schacter, D.L. (2001). *The Seven Sins of Memory*.
8   Burns, D.D. (1980). *Feeling Good: The New Mood Therapy*, Information Australia Group, Melbourne.
9   Burns, D.D. (1980). *Feeling Good: The New Mood Therapy*.
10 Schacter, D.L. (2001). *The Seven Sins of Memory*.
11 Booth, A. (1997). *Improve Your Memory In 21 Days*, Prentice Hall, Sydney, p. 30.
12 This method is a part of neurolinguistic programming (NLP for short) and is based on the idea that different perspectives can alter the intensity of emotional responses to memories.
13 Robbins, A. (1991). *Awaken the Giant Within*, Simon and Schuster, New York. The phrasing used in this quote is from an abridged version on compact disc, CD 1, Sound Ideas, New York.
14 A free booklet on traumatic memory is provided by Veterans Affairs, called 'Posttraumatic stress disorder (PTSD) and war-related stress' by M. Creamer, D. Forbes and G. Devilly. It was written for veterans and their families but is freely available to all the community and provides a general introduction to dealing with traumatic memories in any area of life. To obtain a copy, contact (03) 9496 2922, or email: ncptsd@austin.unimelb.edu or see the website www.ncptsd.unimelb.edu.au
15 Schacter, D.L. (1996). *Searching for Memory: The Brain, the Mind, and the Past*, Basic Books, New York, Chapter 7.
16 Schacter, D.L. (1996). *Searching for Memory: The Brain, the Mind, and the Past*. Susan Greenfield explains that under stress, the neurotransmitter noradrenalin is released and prepares the body for 'fight or flight'; and the neurotransmitter acetycholine quietens the visceral organs when the drama is past. Greenfield, S. (1999). *Brain Power: Working Out the Human Mind*, Element Books, Shaftsbury, Dorset.
17 Schacter, D.L. (2001). *The Seven Sins of Memory*, p. 168. Daniel Schacter describes learning to live with memory's power. In time a person learns to

control the memory instead of being controlled by it. For more details on what is known about traumatic memories, see Chapter 7.

18   Schacter, D.L. (2001). *The Seven Sins of Memory*, p. 178.
19   Schanks, R. (1990). *Tell me a Story*, McMillan Publishing Company, New York.
20   Yates, F.A. (1996). 'The Art of Memory', in McConkey, J. (Ed.) *The Anatomy of Memory: An Anthology*, Oxford University Press, Oxford, p. 15.
21   Yates, F.A. (1996). 'The Art of Memory', p. 17.
22   Yates, F.A. (1996). 'The Art of Memory', p. 11.
23   Two of these currently in libraries and bookshops are: Buzan, T. (1989). *Use Your Head*, BBC Books, London; and Moidel, S. (1992). *Memory Power*, audio tape, Career Track, Boulder.
24   Dickens, Charles (1837). *Pickwick Papers, The Posthumous Papers of the Pickwick Club*, Centennial Edition (1937). Heron Books, London, p. 444–45. The comment is by Mr Weller the elder to Sam Weller.
25   Luria, A.R. (1968). *The Mind of a Mnemonist*, reprinted 1978, Harvard University Press, Cambridge, MA.
26   Baddeley, A. (1996). *Your Memory: A User's Guide*, p. 128. Baddeley is summarising the views of an expert in the field.
27   Schacter, D.L. (2001). *The Seven Sins of Memory*.
28   Squire, L.R. and Kandel, E.R. (1999). *Memory: From Mind to Molecules*, Scientific American Library, New York, p. 71.

Chapter 5
Normal Ageing and Normal Forgetting

1   Dickens, Charles (1839). *Nicholas Nickleby, Hard Times, A Christmas Carol*. From edition published in 1983, Octopus Books, London, p. 193.
2   Belsky, J.K. (1990). *The Psychology of Aging*, 2nd edition, Brooks/Cole Publishing Company, Pacific Grove, California.
3   Balota, D.A., Dolan, P.O. and Duchek, J.M. (2000). 'Memory Changes in Healthy Older Adults', in Tulving, E. and Craik, F.I.M. (Eds), *The Oxford Handbook of Memory*, Oxford University Press, Oxford, pp. 395–409.
4   Balota, D.A., Dolan, P.O., and Duchek, J.M. (2000). 'Memory Changes in Healthy Older Adults'.
5   Schacter, D.L. (1996). *Searching for Memory: The Brain, the Mind, and the Past*, Basic Books, New York.
6   Squire, L.R. and Kandel, E.R. (1999). *Memory: From Mind to Molecules*, Scientific American Library, New York, p. 76.
7   Belsky, J.K. (1990). *The Psychology of Aging*, p. 178–79.
8   Belsky, J.K. (1990). *The Psychology of Aging*.
9   Zarit, S., Cole, K.D. and Guider, R.L. (1981). 'Memory Training Strategies and Subjective Complaints of Memory in the Aged', *The Gerontologist*, Vol. 21, No. 2, pp. 158–64.
10   Belsky, J.K. (1990). *The Psychology of Aging*.

11 Belsky, J.K. (1990). *The Psychology of Aging.*

12 Schacter, D.L. (2001). *The Seven Sins of Memory*, Houghton Mifflin, New York.

13 Schacter, D.L. (1996). *Searching for Memory: The Brain, the Mind, and the Past.*

14 Balota, D.A., Dolan, P.O. and Duchek, J.M. (2000). 'Memory Changes in Healthy Older Adults'.

15 Balota, D.A., Dolan, P.O. and Duchek, J.M. (2000). 'Memory Changes in Healthy Older Adults'.

16 Schacter, D.L. (2001). *The Seven Sins of Memory.*

17 Balota, D.A., Dolan, P.O. and Duchek, J.M. (2000). 'Memory Changes in Healthy Older Adults'.

18 Balota, D.A., Dolan, P.O. and Duchek, J.M. (2000). 'Memory Changes in Healthy Older Adults'.

19 Balota, D.A., Dolan, P.O. and Duchek, J.M. (2000). 'Memory Changes in Healthy Older Adults'.

20 Baddeley, A. (1996). *Your Memory: A User's Guide*, Prion, London.

21 Squire, L.R. and Kandel, E.R. (1999). *Memory: From Mind to Molecules*, p. 206.

22 Schacter, D.L. (1996). *Searching for Memory: The Brain, the Mind, and the Past.*

23 Hampl, P. (1996). 'Memory and Imagination' in McConkey, J. (Ed.), *The Anatomy of Memory: An Anthology*, Oxford University Press, Oxford, pp. 201–11.

24 Barclay, C.R. (1993). 'Remembering Ourselves', in Davies, G.M. and Logie, R.H. (Eds), *Memory in Everyday Life*, North Holland, Amsterdam, pp. 285–309.

25 Smith, R.E. (1993). *Psychology*, West Publishing Company, New York, Chapter 5, pp. 132–65.

26 Casals, P. (1985). 'Joys and Sorrows', quoted in Sampson, A. and Sampson, S. (Eds), *The Oxford Book of Ages*, Oxford University Press, Oxford, p. 176.

27 Andersen-Ranberg, K., Vasegaard, L. and Jeune, B. (2001). 'Dementia is not inevitable: A population-based study of Danish centenarians', *Journal of Gerontology: Psychological Sciences*, Vol. 56B, No. 3, pp. 152–59.

28 Mayer, K.U. et al. (1999). 'What do we know about Old Age and Aging? Conclusions from the Berlin Aging Study', in Baltes, P.B. and Mayer, K.U. (Eds) (1999). *The Berlin Aging Study: Aging from 70 to 100*, Cambridge University Press, Cambridge, pp. 475–519. Mayer and his colleagues argue for recognition that the needs of the old-old are different to those of the young-old. They suggest those who survive into very old age may have physical and psychiatric advantages as well as coping abilities that have allowed them to handle their life circumstances.

29 Levy, B.R., Slade, M.D., Kunkel, S.R. and Kasl, S.V. (2002). 'Longevity Increased by Positive Self-Perceptions of Aging', *Journal of Personality and Social Psychology*, Vol. 83, No. 2, pp. 261–70.

30 Norman Swan's interview was in the Health Report, 22 February 1999 and can be retrieved from www.abc.net.au/rn/talks/8.30/helthrpt/stories/s19117.htm. For more details of the centenarian study, see Perls, T.T., Silver, M.H. and Lauerman, J.F. (2000). *Living to 100: Lessons in Living to Your Maximum Potential at Any Age*, Basic Books, New York, or visit their website at www.med.harvard.edu/program/necs

31 Roden, J. and Langer, E. (1980). 'Aging labels. The decline of control and the fall of self-esteem', *Journal of Social Issues*, Vol. 36, No. 2, pp. 12–29.

32 Johnson, S. (1783), in 'Boswell's Life of Johnson', Vol. 4, p. 181 cited in *The Oxford Dictionary of Quotations*, revised 4th edition, Angela Partington (Ed.) (1996), Oxford University Press, Oxford, p. 376.

33 Baltes, P.B., Mayer, K.U., Helmchen, H. and Steinhagen-Thiessen, E. (1999). 'The Berlin Aging Study (BASE): Sample, Design and Overview of Measures', in Baltes, P.B. and Mayer, K.U. (Eds) (1999). *The Berlin Aging Study: Aging from 70 to 100*, pp. 15–55. Researchers are careful to use the term 'correlation' rather than 'cause' when two events are consistently found to occur together. For example, the sale of ice-creams is correlated with hot days.

34 Sinnott, J.D. (1986). 'Prospective/Intentional and Incidental Everyday Memory: Effects of Age and Passage of Time', *Psychology and Aging*, Vol. 1, No. 2, pp. 110–16.

35 Poon, L.W. (1985). 'Differences in human memory with aging. Nature, causes and clinical implications', in Belsky, J.K. (1990), *The Psychology of Aging*.

36 Schaie, K.W. (1996). *Intellectual Development in Adulthood: The Seattle Longitudinal Study*, Cambridge University Press, Cambridge.

37 Belsky, J.K. (1990). *The Psychology of Aging*.

38 Lyketsos, C.G., Chen, L.S. and Anthony, J. (1999). 'Cognitive decline in adulthood: An 11.5-year follow-up of the Baltimore Epidemiologic Catchment Area Study', *American Journal of Psychiatry*, Vol. 156, No. 1, pp. 58–65. Quote is from p. 58. This point has been made by many researchers.

39 Ekerdt, D.J. (1986). 'The busy ethic. Moral continuity between work and retirement', *Gerontologist*, Vol. 26, pp. 239–44.

40 Belsky, J.K. (1990). *The Psychology of Aging*.

41 Belsky, J.K. (1990). *The Psychology of Aging*.

42 cummings, e. e. (1976). 'old age sticks', in Small, K. (Ed.), *Colour the Wind*, John Wiley, Sydney, p. 61.

43 Belsky, J.K. (1990). *The Psychology of Aging*, p. 47.

44 Belsky, J.K. (1990). *The Psychology of Aging*.

45 Carter, R. (2000). *Mapping the Mind*, Phoenix, London.

46 Jennings, C.R. and Jones, N.S. (2001). 'Presbyacusis', *The Journal of Laryngology and Otology*, Vol. 115, pp. 171–78.

47 For more details of glaucoma, see the website at www.glaucoma.org

48 The syndrome was named after a Swiss naturalist whose grandfather had such visions. Ockham's Razor 'Old age and dementia' was presented by Professor John Bradshaw on 4 September, 1999. The transcript is available from the Radio National website.

49 Belsky J.K. (1990). *The Psychology of Aging*, p. 15.

50 Simonton, D.K. (1990). 'Creativity in the Later Years: Optimistic Prospects for Achievement', *Symposium*, Vol. 30, No. 5, pp. 626–31.

51 Belsky, J.K. (1990). *The Psychology of Aging*.

52 Schacter, D.L. (1996). *Searching for Memory: The Brain, the Mind, and the Past*.

53 Fuster, J.M. (1997). 'Network Memory', *Trends in Neuroscience*, Vol. 20, No. 10, pp. 451–59.

54 Selkoe, D.J. (1993). 'Aging Brain, Aging Mind', in *Mind and Brain: Readings from Scientific American Magazine*, W.H. Freeman and Company, New York.

55 Hippocampal neurons redrawn from Selkoe, D.J. (1993). 'Aging Brain, Aging Mind' in *Mind and Brain: Readings from Scientific American Magazine*, p. 105.

Chapter 6
Normal Memory Loss or Alzheimer's?

1 Schacter, D.L. (1996). *Searching for Memory: The Brain, the Mind, and the Past*, Basic Books, New York, p. 285.

2 Technically it is a misuse of the terminology to say that someone 'has Alzheimer's disease' since the diagnosis is unsure while they are living. Hence we will use the phrases 'people with probable Alzheimer's disease' or 'people with dementia of the Alzheimer's type (DAT)'. DAT is currently the preferred diagnostic term. See Gruetzner, H. (1997). *Alzheimer's: The Complete Guide for Families and Loved Ones*, John Wiley & Sons, New York.

3 Gruetzner, H. (1997). *Alzheimer's: The Complete Guide for Families and Loved Ones*.

4 Baddeley, A. (1996). *Your Memory: A User's Guide*, Prion, London.

5 The regions most affected early in Alzheimer's are the input region to the hippocampus called the entorhinal cortex and a second region called CA1 in the hippocampus. As the disease progresses it affects areas involved in attention, the temporal cortex and other brain areas. By contrast, the regions most affected in age-related memory decline occur in the output regions of the hippocampus called the dentate gyrus and the subiculum. See Gruetzner, H. (1997). *Alzheimer's: The Complete Guide for Families and Loved Ones*, Chapter 14, pp. 205–33; Squire, L.R. and Kandel, E.R. (1999). *Memory: From Mind to Molecules*, Scientific American Library, New York, pp. 206–11.

6 Alzheimer's Association NSW (1997). 'The Dementias', in *Help Notes*, p. 4, available from www.alznsw.asn.au. Many sources address differences between normal ageing and dementia, such as the video *Forgetfulness: Normal or Dementia?* Address for 1996 National Alzheimer's Week by Dr Wayne Reid, Research Fellow Neuropsychologist, Department of Geriatric Medicine, Concord Hospital (available from the Alzheimer's Association).

7 Gruetzner, H. (1997). *Alzheimer's: The Complete Guide for Families and Loved Ones*.

8 Creasy, H. and Brodaty, H. (1999). 'Research Briefs', *InTouch*, Winter, p. 7.

9 Estimated rates of Alzheimer's disease differ widely. The figures we give are typical, and are from two sources: The Baltimore Longitudinal Study of Aging, reported in Kawas, C., Gray, S., Brookmeyer, R., Fozard, J. and Zonderman,

A. (2000). 'Age-specific incidence rates of Alzheimer's disease', *Neurology*, Vol. 54, pp. 2072–77; and a population in Boston, Mass. reported in Hebet, L.E. et al. (1995). 'Age–specific incidence of Alzheimer's disease in a community population', *Journal American Medical Association*, Vol. 273, No. 17, pp. 1354–59. For a meta-analysis of incidence rates, see Jorm, A.F. and Jolly, D. (1998). 'The incidence of dementia: a meta-analysis', *Neurology*, Vol. 51, No. 3, pp. 728–33.

10 Jorm, A. (2001). 'Dementia: A major health problem for Australia, position paper 1', pp. 1–5. Available from the Alzheimer's Association Australia web page.

11 Prevalence rates for Australia, Europe and USA vary on average from 1.4 per cent in the age group 64–69, rising to 23.6 per cent for the age group over 85. For a table of results showing averages for all ages, see the Alzheimer's Disease International Fact Sheet No. 3: 'The Prevalence of Dementia', available online from www.alz.co.uk

12 There is concern among many people that if they live long enough they will eventually suffer from dementia. As we note in the text, the risks do increase up to the age of 90, but different studies report prevalence rates that vary widely. Sample sizes and methods probably account for much of this difference, as well as differences in regional populations and lifestyles. Some studies show that the risks may even decline in the nineties. Among the oldest old, one study showed that dementia is common but not inevitable for 100 year olds, with an estimated 25–37 per cent of centenarians in Denmark showing no signs of dementia. The study is reported in Andersen-Ranberg, K., Vasegaard, L. and Jeune, B. (2001). 'Dementia is not inevitable: a population-based study of Danish centenarians', *Journal of Gerontology: Psychological Sciences*, Vol. 56B, No. 3, pp. 152–59.

13 Alzheimer's Society, 'Statistics about dementia'. Available online from the Alzheimer's Society UK web page at www.alzheimers.org.uk/about/statistics

14 For more information on regional differences, see the Alzheimer's Disease International Fact Sheet No. 3. 'The Prevalence of Dementia', available online from www.alz.co.uk

15 For a summary of these issues, see the Alzheimer's Association information page, 'Am I at Risk of developing Alzheimer's disease?' October 2001, available online from www.alzheimers.org.uk.

16 Lindenberger, U. and Reischies, F.M. (1999). 'Limits and potentials of intellectual functioning in old age', in Baltes, P.B. and Mayer, K.U. (Eds). *The Berlin Aging Study*, Cambridge University Press, Cambridge, MA, pp. 329–59.

17 Boden, Christine (1998). *Who will I be when I die?* HarperCollins Religious, Melbourne, p. 167.

18 Boden, Christine (1998). *Who will I be when I die?* p. 153.

19 Greiner, P.A., Snowden, D.A. and Greiner, L.H. (1996). 'The Relationship of self-rated function and self-rated health to concurrent functional ability, functional decline, and mortality: Findings from the Nun Study', *Journal of Gerontology: Social Sciences*, Vol. 51B, No. 5. pp. S234–41.

20 West, L. (2001). '*Early Stage Dementia: Reassurance for sufferers and carers*', Hodder Headline Australia, Sydney, p. 16.

21 The diagnosis of Alzheimer's disease requires assessment by a clinician skilled in diagnosing dementia, using the criteria established by the National Institute of Neurological and Communicative Disorders and Stroke – Alzheimer's Disease and Related Disorders Association (NINCDS-ADRDA). The diagnosis of *probable* Alzheimer's disease is supported by: progressive deterioration of specific cognitive functions such as language (aphasia), motor skills (apraxia) and perception (agnosia); impaired activities of daily living and altered patterns of behaviour; family history of similar disorders, particularly if confirmed neuropathologically, see *Medical Journal of Australia*, Vol. 172, 3 April, 2000, p. 339.

22 Herman Buschke's test involves multiple encoding and cued recall, which presents little difficulty for normally ageing people, but is very difficult for those with DAT. A simple description of the test is given by Daniel Schacter (2001) in *The Seven Sins of Memory*, p. 21. For a more complete description, see the chapter by Lindenberger, U. and Reischies, F.M. (1999). 'Limits and potentials of intellectual functioning in old age', in Baltes, P.B. and Mayer, K.U. (Eds), *The Berlin Aging Study*, especially pages 348–51.

23 Folstein, M.F., Folstein S.E. and McHugh P.R. (1975). 'Mini-Mental State – a practical method for grading the cognitive state of patients for the clinician', *Journal of Psychiatric Research*, Vol. 12, pp. 189–98.

24 Lyketsos, C.G., Chen, L.S. and Anthony, J.C. (1999). 'Cognitive decline in adulthood: An 11.5-year follow-up of the Baltimore epidemiologic catchment area study', *American Journal of Psychiatry*, Vol. 156, No. 1, pp. 58–65.

25 The Silly Sentences test examples are from Baddeley, A. (1996). *Your Memory: A User's Guide*, p. 177–78.

26 Tulving, E. and Craik, F.I.M. (2000). *The Oxford Handbook of Memory*, Oxford University Press, Oxford, Preface, p. vii.

27 Alzheimer's Society (2002). 'Aluminium and Alzheimer's disease', *Information sheet 406*, June. Available online from www.alzheimers.org.uk

28 For more details on CAT scans, see Gazzaniga, M.S., Ivry, R.B. and Mangun, G.R. (1998). *Cognitive Neuroscience: The Biology of the Mind*, W.W. Norton & Company, New York.

29 Carter, R. (2000). *Mapping the Mind*, Phoenix, London; Greenfield, S. (1999). *Brain Power: Working Out the Human Mind*, Element Books, Shaftsbury, Dorset.

30 News scan (2002). 'Scanning for Dementia', *Scientific American*, Vol. 287, No. 5, p. 13. The radioactive tracer is called FDDNP.

31 Redrawn from Fischbach, G.D. (1993). 'Mind and Brain', in *Mind and Brain: Readings from Scientific American Magazine*, W.H. Freeman and Company, New York, p. 13.

32 Gazzaniga, M.S., Ivry, R.B. and Mangun, G.R. (1998). *Cognitive Neuroscience: The Biology of the Mind.*

33 Greenfield, S. (2000). *Brain Story*, BBC Worldwide, London.

34 Boden, Christine (1998). *Who will I be when I die?* HarperCollins Religious, Melbourne, pp. 58–59.

35 Greenfield, S. (1999). *Brain Power: Working Out the Human Mind.*

36 Gruetzner, H. (1997). *Alzheimer's: The Complete Guide for Families and Loved Ones.*

37 Panegyres, P.K., Connor, C., Liebeck, T., Goldblatt, J., Walpole, I. and Harrop, K. (2000). 'Education, counselling, support' in *Medical Journal of Australia*, 3 April, p. 339.

38 Creasy, H. and Brodaty, H. (Hon. Medical Advisers to The Alzheimer's Association NSW). (2001). 'Research Briefs', *In Touch*.

39 Greenfield, S. (1999). *Brain Power: Working Out the Human Mind*, p. 135.

40 *Eighth International Conference on Alzheimer's Disease and Related Disorders*, Stockholm, Sweden, 2002. For further details, see the website at: www.alz.org/internationalconference

41 Martindale, D. (2002). 'Peeling Plaque', *Scientific American*, Vol. 287, No. 5, pp. 12–13.

42 Pinel, J.P.J. (1997). *Biopsychology*, 3rd edition, Allyn & Bacon, Boston.

43 There are many theories of the causes of Alzheimer's disease. For more details of the theory we present here and the genetic risk factors in the early and late forms, an excellent summary is given in Squire, L.R. and Kandel, E.R. (1999). *Memory: From Mind to Molecules*, pp. 206–11.

44 The gene that codes for the protein apolipoprotein E (ApoE) on chromosome 19 is involved in cholesterol metabolism. Three different alleles of this gene are known, and people with one of the forms (ApoE4) have a higher chance of developing the disease. If a person has two copies of the allele (one from each parent) they have an even higher chance. The other gene of interest codes for the protein A2M on chromosome 12 and is also involved in clean-up operations. For more details, see Squire, L.R. and Kandel, E.R. (1999). *Memory: From Mind to Molecules*, pp. 208–10.

45 Kivipelto, M. (2002). *Eighth International Conference on Alzheimer's Disease and Related Disorders*, Stockholm, Sweden. Several other studies have also shown a relationship between high cholesterol in midlife and late onset Alzheimer's. For example, see Kivipelto M., et al. (2001). 'Midlife vascular risk factors and Alzheimer's disease in later life: longitudinal, population-based study', *British Medical Journal*, Vol. 322, pp. 1447–51.

46 Estimates of the genetic component of Alzheimer's disease vary widely. For example, Gazzaniga, Ivry and Mangun, in Gazzaniga, M.S., Ivry, R.B. and Mangun, G.R. (1988). *Cognitive Neuroscience: The Biology of the Mind*, p. 89, state that only 5 per cent of cases are clearly related to a genetic component and that in late onset Alzheimer's (that is, after the age of 65) the vast majority of people had no family history of the condition. However, Pinel, in Pinel, J.P.J. (1997). *Biopsychology*, p. 143, cites the higher figure of 50 per cent for people who have an immediate family member with the disease and survive into their nineties. Squire and Kandel, in Squire, L.R. and Kandel, E.R. (1999). *Memory: From Mind to Molecules*, p. 209, suggest that as many as 30 per cent of people with the late onset form may carry a mutated version of the A2M gene. Given

the ages involved, many people die of natural causes before Alzheimer's symptoms appear. Even the practical consequences of genetic risk factors are as yet unclear. Although ApoE4 is known to be a risk factor for developing Alzheimer's disease, the benefits of ApoE genotyping are yet to be determined.

Chapter 7
Maintaining Health for Vintage Memories

1   Wahlqvist, M. (1999). From an address given at an Australian Nutrition Foundation seminar on 'Nutrition and Healthy Ageing', *COTA News*, Council on the Ageing (NSW) (COTA), March, p. 8.
2   Kramer, A.F. et al. (1999). 'Ageing, fitness and neurocognitive function', *Nature*, Vol. 400, No. 6743, pp. 418–19.
3   Yaffe, K., Barnes, D., Nevitt, M., Lui, L. and Covinnsky, K. (2001). 'A Prospective Study of Physical Activity and Cognitive Decline in Elderly Women', *Archives of Internal Medicine*, Vol. 161, pp. 1703–08.
4   Royal Prince Alfred Hospital, Sydney (2002). 'Module 3: Movement is activity and activity is exercise', in *Bodylines: Weight Management Program for Women*, Metabolism and Obesity services.
5   Studies in the US have shown that the fear of falling confines older people to their homes. However, Julie Halbert and Paul Finucane list 11 major benefits of exercise which include cardiorespiratory fitness and say that the 'benefits will outweigh the risks for most elderly people providing sensible precautions are taken'. See Halbert, J. and Finucane, P. (2001). 'Exercise and Elderly People', in *Australian Doctor*, 15 June, p. 2.
6   Nelson, M. (2001). *Strong Women Stay Young*, Lothian Aurum Press, Port Melbourne.
7   Royal Prince Alfred Hospital, Sydney (2002). 'Module 3: Movement is activity and activity is exercise', in *Bodylines, Weight Management Program for Women*, Metabolism and Obesity services. See also, Halbert, J. and Finucane, P. (2001). 'Exercise and Elderly People'.
8   Schacter, D.L. (1996). *Searching for Memory: The Brain, the Mind, and the Past*, Basic Books, New York; Carter, R. (2000). *Mapping the Mind*, Phoenix, London.
9   McClelland, J.L, McNaughton, B.L. and O'Reilly, R.C. (1995). 'Why there are complementary learning systems in hippocampus and neocortex: Insights from the successes and failures of connectionist models of learning and memory', *Psychological Review*, Vol. 102, pp. 419–57.
10 Cheour, M. et al. (2002). 'Psychobiology: Speech sounds learned by sleeping newborns', *Nature*, Vol. 415, pp. 599–600.
11 Greenfield, S. (1999). *Brain Power: Working Out the Human Mind*, Element Books, Shaftsbury, Dorset; Lewey, A.J., Ahmed, S. and Sack, R.L. (1996). 'Phase shifting in the human circadian clock using melatonin', in *Behavioural Brain Research*, Vol. 73, pp. 131–34.

12 Smith, R.E. (1993). *Psychology*, West Publishing Company, New York.

13 Zhdanova, I.V. et al. (1995). 'Sleep-inducing effects of low doses of melatonin ingested in the evening', *Clinical Pharmacology and Therapeutics*, Vol. 57, No. 5, pp. 552–58.

14 Curran, H.V. (2000). 'Psychopharmacological Perspectives on Memory', in Tulving, E. and Craik F.I.M. (Eds). *The Oxford Handbook of Memory*, Oxford University Press, Oxford, p. 540.

15 David Morawetz is a clinical psychologist and counsellor who developed the *Sleep Better Without Drugs* booklet and audio tape (1994) available from the Sleep Better Hotline on 1 800 066 044.

16 Job, E. (1991). *Keeping Memory Keen and Fending off Forgetfulness.* Booklet developed for a Continuing Education program at The University of Queensland.

17 Morawetz, D. (1994). *Sleep Better Without Drugs*, p. 32.

18 Davies, S.R. (Ed.) (2000). 'Supplement', *The Medical Journal of Australia*, Vol. 173, 6 November, p. S109.

19 Cohen, S. and Miller, G.E. (2001). 'Stress, Immunity, and Susceptibility to Upper Respiratory Infection', in Ader, R., Felton, D.L. and Cohen, N. (Eds). *Psychoneuroimmunology*, 3rd edition, Vol. 2, Chapter 56, Academic Press, New York. pp. 499–509.

20 Smith, R.E. (1993). *Psychology*.

21 Levy, B.R., Slade, M.D., Kunkel, S.R. and Kasl, S.V. (2002). 'Longevity Increased by Positive Self-Perceptions of Aging', *Journal of Personality and Social Psychology*, Vol. 83, No. 2, pp. 261–70. The study is one of the few that predict survival on positive factors. Most studies have been done on negative factors such as disease, injury and cognitive decline and very few on the contributions that positive self perceptions may make to longevity.

22 Manning, C.A., Hall, J.L. and Gold, P.E. (1990). 'Glucose effects on memory and other neurophysiological tests in elderly humans', *Psychological Science*, Vol. 1, No. 5, September, pp. 307–11.

23 Pratchett, T. (1993). *Men at Arms*, Corgi, London, p. 173.

24 Savige, G., Wahlqvist, M., Lee, D. and Snelson, B. (2001). *ageFIT: Fitness and nutrition for an independent future*, Pan Macmillan, Sydney.

25 Research into the role of the different types of fat is ongoing, and has more subtleties than we can mention here. For a readable summary of the different types of fats, see Chapter 18 'Macronutrients' in Savige, G., Wahlqvist, M., Lee, D. and Snelson, B. (2001). *ageFIT: Fitness and nutrition for an independent future*, pp. 166–85.

26 Epidemiology studies interactions between components of disease and environmental factors, and controlling health problems over the population as a whole.

27 Willett, W.C. and Stampfer, M.J. (2003). 'Rebuilding the food pyramid', *Scientific American*, Vol. 288, No. 1, pp. 52–59. They go on to explain that rapid increases in blood sugar levels can stimulate a large increase in insulin, the hormone that directs glucose to the muscles, which in turn can cause a rapid drop in blood sugar, even sending it below baseline levels. Refined carbohydrates can also

have negative effects by lowering good cholesterol and raising triglycerides, the component molecules of fat.

28 Willett, W.C. and Stampfer, M.J. (2003). 'Rebuilding the food pyramid', p. 55.
29 Willett, W.C. and Stampfer, M.J. (2003). 'Rebuilding the food pyramid'.
30 CSIRO is Australia's Commonwealth Science and Industry Research Organisation.
31 See for example, Kouris-Blazos, A. (2002). 'Dietary advice and food guidance systems', Chapter 38 in Wahlqvist, M.L. (Ed.) *Food and Nutrition Australasia, Asia and the Pacific*, 2nd edition, Allen & Unwin, Sydney, pp. 531–57.
32 This food pyramid is a simplified version of Willett and Stampfer's 'New Food Pyramid' in 'Rebuilding the food pyramid', p. 55.
33 *Stedman's Medical Dictionary*.
34 Savige, G., Wahlqvist, M., Lee, D. and Snelson, B. (2001). *ageFIT: Fitness and nutrition for an independent future*.
35 World Health Organisation (1996). Quoted in *COTA News*, March 1999, p. 8.
36 Coombes, J.S. (2002). 'Antioxidants and Ageing', in *Ageing Research: A cross-disciplinary view*, University of Queensland Centre for Human Ageing, Colloquium Series 2001, Brisbane, pp. 1–8.
37 For foods rich in antioxidants see Saxelby, C. (2001). *Nutrition for the Healthy Heart*, Hardie Grant Books, South Yarra, Victoria.
38 Kouris-Blazos, A. (2002). 'Dietary advice and food guidance systems'.
39 Savige, G., Wahlqvist, M., Lee, D. and Snelson, B. (2001). *ageFIT: Fitness and nutrition for an independent future*.
40 Coombes, J.S. (2001). 'Antioxidants and Ageing' in *Ageing Research: A cross-disciplinary view*.
41 Pinel, J.P.J. (1997). *Biopsychology*, 3rd edition, Allyn & Bacon, Boston. p. 241.
42 Stanton, R. (1999). *Vitamins: What they do and what they don't do*. Allen & Unwin, Sydney. Stanton also warns of the dangers of taking too many supplements as antioxidants, because the body's antioxidant defence system is finely balanced and too much can cause biomolecular damage.
43 Coombes, J.S. (2001). 'Antioxidants and Ageing', in *Ageing Research: A cross-disciplinary view*.
44 Recommended dosages of vitamin E vary widely in the popular press. Neurology professors Guy McKhann and Marilyn Albert recommend 1000 units (670 milligrams) daily for its preventative potential. McKhann, G. and Albert, M. (2002). *Keep Your Brain Young*, John Wiley, New York.
45 A study that found DNA changes in volunteers taking supplements of 500 milligrams of vitamin C is reported in Stanton, R. (1999). *Vitamins: What they do and what they don't do*.
46 People who eat more fruits and vegetables that are rich in vitamins have been shown to have lower risks of cancer, but supplements can have different effects, and higher risks of cancer were found in smokers taking beta-carotene supplements. See studies by Wang, X.D. and Russell, R.M. (1999). 'Procarcinogenic and anticarcinogenic effects of betacarotene', *Nutrition Reviews*, Vol. 57. No. 9I, pp. 263–72.

47 Savige, G., Wahlqvist, M., Lee, D. and Snelson, B. (2001). *ageFIT: Fitness and nutrition for an independent future.*

48 Mackenzie, J. (Ed.) (2001). 'Alternative Therapies: Do they Help?', *Choice*, September, p. 18.

49 McKhann, G. and Albert, M. (2002). *Keep Your Brain Young.*

50 Squire, L.R. and Kandel, E.R. (1999). *Memory: From Mind to Molecules*, Scientific American Library, New York, p. 205.

51 Gold, P.E., Cahill, L., and Wenk, G.L. (2003). 'The lowdown on Gingko Biloba', *Scientific American*, Vol. 288, No. 2, pp. 69–73. See also DeFeudis, F.V. and Drieu, K. (2000). 'Ginkgo Biloba Extract (EGb 761) and CNS Functions: Basic Studies and Clinical Applications', *Current Drug Targets*, Vol. 1, p. 25–58.

52 Rigney, U., Kimber, S. and Hindmarch, I. (1999). 'The effects of acute doses of standardized Ginko Biloba extract on memory and psychomotor performance in volunteers', *Phytotherapy Research*, Vol. 13, pp. 408–15.

53 The background of how thiamine came to be accepted in bread but not in beer is told by A. Stewart Truswell in 'Report to ANZFA on the thiamin status of Australians and the potential health impacts of adjustments to dietary thiamine intake as a result of changes to mandatory fortification requirements in food regulation'. Available from the Food Standards Australia New Zealand website: www.fsanz.gov.au

54 ABC Radio National program (2001). 'Background Briefing', 30 September.

55 Briggs, D.R. and Lennard, L.B. (2002). 'Food law and regulation', Chapter 9 in Wahlqvist, M.L. (Ed.), *Food and Nutrition Australasia, Asia and the Pacific*, 2nd edition, Allen & Unwin, Sydney, pp. 137–51.

56 'Food fight', *Australian Doctor*, 18 May 2001, pp. 40–44, quoting *British Medical Journal*, (2000), Vol. 320, pp. 861–64.

57 Stanton, R. (1999). *Vitamins: What they do and what they don't do.*

58 Mackenzie, J. (Ed.) (2002). 'And the logo goes to …', *Choice*, November, pp. 12–15; Mackenzie, J. (Ed.) (2003). 'Food labels uncut', *Choice*, August, pp. 8–13.

59 Creasy, H. and Brodaty, H. (2001). 'Research Briefs', *InTouch*, Winter, p. 7.

60 Briggs, D.R. and Lennard, L.B. (2002). 'Food law and regulation'.

61 The lack of standardisation in alternative medicines is made in *every* nutrition book we consulted. See, for example, Mackenzie, J. (Ed.) (2001). 'Alternative Therapies: Do they Help?', *Choice*, September, pp. 18–24; the Medline website: www.ncbi.nim.nih.gov/PubMed; or McKhann, G., and Albert, M. (2002). *Keep Your Brain Young.*

62 Food Standards Australia and New Zealand has a very useful website with advice on a wide range of food issues: www.fsanz.gov.au

63 Mackenzie, J. (Ed.) (2001). 'Alternative Therapies: Do they Help?', *Choice*, September, pp. 18–24.

64 Savige, G., Wahlqvist, M., Lee, D. and Snelson, B. (2001). *ageFIT: Fitness and nutrition for an independent future.*

65 Kurth, T., et al. (2002). 'Body mass index and the risk of stroke in men', *Archives of Internal Medicine*, Vol. 162, No. 22, pp. 2557–62.

66 Australian Bureau of Statistics. 'Australian Social Trends (2002): Health – Mortality and Morbidity: Cardiovascular Disease: 20th Century Trends.'

67 Cervilla, J. A., Prince, M., and Mann, A. (2000). 'Smoking, drinking, and incident cognitive impairment: a cohort community based study included in the Gospel Oak project', *Journal of Neurology, Neurosurgery and Psychiatry*, Vol. 68, pp. 622–26.

68 Quitters' Page: www.quitnow.info.au/quitterspage.html

69 Klatsky, A.L. (2003). 'Drink to your health?' *Scientific American*, Vol. 288, No. 2, pp. 63–69.

70 These figures are from Saxelby, C. (2001), *Nutrition for the Healthy Heart*. The recommendations of the National Health and Medical Research Council are no more than two standard drinks per day for women and four for men, and some alcohol-free days per week, with reduced amounts for older people as the body's tolerance decreases with age. An Australian standard drink contains 10 grams of alcohol, and is approximately a nip of spirits (30 ml), a small glass of wine (100 ml) or a middy/pot of beer (285 ml). 'Australian Alcohol Guidelines', is available from www.alcoholguidelines.gov.au/standard.htm

71 Carter, R. (2000). *Mapping the Mind*.

72 Baddeley, A. (1996). *Your Memory: A User's Guide*, Prion, London.

73 Greenfield, S. (1999). *Brain Power: Working Out the Human Mind*.

74 Belsky, J.K. (1990). *The Psychology of Aging*, 2nd edition, Brooks/Cole Publishing Company, Pacific Grove, California.

75 Greenfield, S. (2000). *Brain Story*, BBC Worldwide, London, pp. 128–35.

76 *Australian Doctor* (25 May 2001) attributes the sense of well being to 'physical and psychiatric advantages as well as coping strategies that helped them handle life's circumstances' – a 'hardy survivor effect' (quoting the *Journal of Gerontology*, 2001,Vol. 56, pp. 111–18).

77 Greenfield, S. (2000). *Brain Story*.

78 Ader, R., Felton, D. L. and Cohen, N. (Eds). (2001). *Psychoneuroimmunology*, 3rd edition, Vol. 2, Academic Press, New York. See especially the chapters by Biondi, M. 'Effects of Stress on Immune Functions: An Overview', Chapter 39, pp. 189–226; and Solomon, G. F. and Morley, J.E. 'Psychoneuroimmunology and Aging', Chapter 67, pp. 701–17.

79 Wilkes, G.A. and Krebs, W.A. (1982). *Collins Concise English Dictionary*, Australian Edition. Collins, Sydney.

80 Greenfield, S. (1999). *Brain Power: Working Out the Human Mind*.

81 Dhabhar, F.S. and McEwen, B. (2001). 'Bidirectional effects of stress and glucocorticoid hormones on immune function: Possible explanations for paradoxical observations', Chapter 10 in Ader, R., Felton, D. L. and Cohen, N. (Eds). *Psychoneuroimmunology*, 3rd edition, Vol. 1. Academic Press, New York. pp. 301–30.

82 Biondi, M. (2001). 'Effects of Stress on Immune Functions: An Overview', p. 217.

83 Smith, R.E. (1993). *Psychology*, p. 92.

84 Dhabhar, F.S. and McEwen, B. (2001). 'Bidirectional effects of stress and glucocorticoid hormones on immune function: Possible explanations for paradoxical observations'.
85 Biondi, M. (2001). 'Effects of Stress on Immune Functions: An Overview'.
86 Solomon, G.F. and Morley, J.E. (2001). 'Psychoneuroimmunology and Aging'.
87 Smith, R.E. (1993). *Psychology*.
88 This quote is attributed in a variety of forms to William James or James Truslow Adams.

Chapter 8
The Brain in Action

1 Damasio, A.R. (1994). *Descartes' Error: Emotion, Reason and the Human Brain*, Avon Books, New York, p. 90.
2 Greenfield, S. (2000). *Brain Story*, BBC Worldwide, London.
3 Greenfield, S. (1999). *Brain Power: Working Out the Human Mind*, Element Books, Shaftsbury, Dorset.
4 Rupp, R. (1998). *Committed to Memory: How we remember and why we forget*, Crown, New York.
5 Greenfield, S. (2000). *Brain Story*, See also Pinel, J.P.J. (1997). *Biopsychology*, 3rd edition, Allyn & Bacon, Boston.
6 Greenfield, S. (2000). *Brain Story*.
7 Pinel, J.P.J. (1997). *Biopsychology*.
8 Greenfield, S. (1999). *Brain Power: Working Out the Human Mind*.
9 Pinel, J.P.J. (1997). *Biopsychology*.
10 Pinel, J.P.J. (1997). *Biopsychology*.
11 Lego® is a trademark of the Lego Group of companies.
12 Squire, L.R. and Kandel E.R. (1999). *Memory: From Mind to Molecules*, Scientific American Library, New York.
13 Pinel, J.P.J. (1997). *Biopsychology*; see also Squire, L.R. and Kandel, E.R. (1999). *Memory: From Mind to Molecules*.
14 Greenfield, S. (2000). *Brain Story*.
15 Squire, L.R. and Kandel, E.R. (1999). *Memory: From Mind to Molecules*.
16 Squire, L.R. and Kandel, E.R. (1999). *Memory: From Mind to Molecules*.
17 Pinel, J.P.J. (1997). *Biopsychology*; Greenfield, S. (2000). *Brain Story*; Squire, L.R. and Kandel, E.R. (1999). *Memory: From Mind to Molecules*; Carter, R. (2000). *Mapping the Mind*, Phoenix, London.
18 Curran, V.H. (2000). 'Psychopharmacological perspectives on memory', Chapter 33 in Tulving, E. and Craik, F.I.M. (Eds), *The Oxford Handbook of Memory*, Oxford University Press, Oxford, pp. 539–54.
19 Greenfield, S. (2000). *Brain Story*.
20 Carter, R. (2000). *Mapping the Mind*; Greenfield, S. (2000). *Brain Story*.
21 Carter, R. (2000). *Mapping the Mind*; Greenfield, S. (2000). *Brain Story*.

22 Carter, R. (2000). *Mapping the Mind*.

23 Greenfield, S. (2000). *Brain Story*.

24 Carter, R. (2000). *Mapping the Mind*.

25 Carter, R. (2000). *Mapping the Mind*.

26 Fuster, J.M. (1997). 'Network Memory', *Trends in Neuroscience*, Vol. 20, No. 10, pp. 451–59.

27 Carter, R. (2000). *Mapping the Mind*, p. 22.

28 Fischbach, G.D. (1993). 'Mind and Brain', in *Mind and Brain: Readings from Scientific American Magazine*, pp. 1–14.

29 Carter, R. (2000). *Mapping the Mind*.

30 Greenfield, S. (1999). *Brain Power: Working Out the Human Mind*, p. 17.

31 From the 1920s to the 1950s, Karl Lashley, professor of psychology at Harvard University conducted experiments on rats to see which areas and how much of their brains he could surgically remove before the rats forgot how to run a maze, which they had previously learned thoroughly. He found that no single area in the cortex was critical, and that more errors were made in re-learning as the extent of the damage increased. However, Lashley did not remove the deeper structures including the hippocampus, which is now thought to be crucial for spatial memory. The rats would remember how to run the maze, but other abilities would have been damaged. There is a popular misconception that we only use a small fraction of our brains, which is quite wrong. We use all aspects of our brains, each region having a specialised role that contributes to many different tasks. Squire, L.R. and Kandel, E.R. (1999). *Memory: From Mind to Molecules*.

32 Squire, L.R. and Kandel, E.R. (1999). *Memory: From Mind to Molecules*, p. 10.

33 Greenfield, S. (2000). *Brain Story*.

34 Greenfield, S. (1999). *Brain Power: Working Out the Human Mind*.

35 Schacter, D.L. (2001). *The Seven Sins of Memory*, Houghton Mifflin, New York; Carter, R. (2000). *Mapping the Mind*.

36 Ramachandran, V.S. and Blakeslee, S. (1998). *Phantoms in the Brain: Probing the Mysteries of the Human Mind*, William Morrow, New York.

37 Booth, A. (1997). *Improve Your Memory in 21 Days*, Prentice Hall, Sydney. p. 55.

38 Carter, R. (2000), *Mapping the Mind*.

39 Damasio, A.R. (1994). *Descartes' Error: Emotion, Reason and the Human Brain*.

40 Squire, L.R. and Kandel E.R. (1999). *Memory: From Mind to Molecules*.

41 Carter, R. (2000). *Mapping the Mind*.

42 Schacter, D.L. (1996). *Searching for Memory: The Brain, the Mind and the Past*, Basic Books, New York.

43 Squire, L.R. and Kandel E.R. (1999). *Memory: From Mind to Molecules*.

44 West, R. and Alain, C. (2000). 'Evidence for the transient nature of a neural system supporting goal-directed action', *Cerebral Cortex*, Vol. 10, No. 8, pp. 748–52.

45 For a review on the differences between anxiety and conditioned fear responses, see 'Anxiety disorders treatment target: Amygdala Circuitry' at the website www.nimh.nih.gov/events/pranxst.cfm

46 LeDoux, J. (1994). 'Emotion, Memory and the Brain', *Scientific American*, Vol. 270, No. 6, pp. 50–57.
47 Squire, L.R. and Kandel, E.R. (1999). *Memory: From Mind to Molecules*.
48 Squire, L.R. and Kandel, E.R. (1999). *Memory: From Mind to Molecules*.
49 Gleick, J. (1999). *Faster: The Acceleration of Just About Everything*, Little, Brown and Co., London, p. 265.
50 Squire, L.R. and Kandel, E.R. (1999). *Memory: From Mind to Molecules*.
51 Damasio, A.R. and Damasio, H. (1993). 'Brain and Language', in *Mind and Brain, Readings from Scientific American*, W.H. Freeman and Company, New York, pp. 61–65.
52 Carter, R. (2000). *Mapping the Mind*.
53 Pinel, J.P.J. (1997). *Biopsychology*.
54 Specifically, the part of the hippocampus is the dentate gyrus, part of the output region of the hippocampus. See Squire, L.R. and Kandel E.R. (1999). *Memory: From Mind to Molecules*.
55 Redrawn by Nic Geard from Kemperman, G. and Gage, F.H. (2002). 'New nerve cells for the adult brain', *Scientific American*, Vol. 287, No. 8, pp. 38–44.
56 Kemperman, G. and Gage, F.H. (2002). 'New nerve cells for the adult brain'.
57 This is a key message in LeDoux, J. (2002). *Synaptic Self: How Our Brains Become Who We Are*, Viking, New York.

Chapter 9
Lifelong Memory, Lifelong Learning

1   Squire, L.R. and Kandel E.R. (1999). *Memory: From Mind to Molecules*, Scientific American Library, New York, Preface, p. ix.
2   Greenfield, S. (2000). *Brain Story*, BBC Worldwide, London, p. 197.
3   The library of Unseen University in Terry Pratchett's fantastic 'Disc World' series works like this.
4   H.G. Wells (1937). Quoted in Gleick, J. (1999). *Faster: The Acceleration of Just About Everything*, Little Brown and Co., London, pp. 254–55.
5   This quote is apochryphal but serves to illustrate the vast changes that have occurred within living memory. From: www.ox.compsoc.net/~swhite/history/timeline-QUOTES.html#77
6   Pobjie, L. (2002). 'Computers', *North Shore Times*, 7 August.
7   In 1999, the size of the World Wide Web was estimated to be 800,000,000 pages. The extraordinary thing is that such a huge amount of information can be accessed very rapidly. The search engine with the largest coverage was estimated to index about 38 per cent of those documents. Digging further into the web analogy for memory, there is estimated to be ten times as much information again (called 'dark matter' in analogy to physics), which is not directly accessible to search engines. See Albert R., Jeong, H. and Barabasi, A.L. (1999). 'Internet: Diameter of the World Wide Web', *Nature*, Vol. 401, pp. 130–31.

8   Damasio, A.R. (1994). *Descartes' Error: Emotion, Reason and the Human Brain*. Avon Books, New York.
9   Halal, W.E. and Liebowitz, J. (1994). 'Telelearning: The Multimedia Revolution in Education', *The Futurist*, November–December, p. 21.
10 Gleick, J. (1999). *Faster: The Acceleration of Just About Everything*.
11 Jeanette Harper is an artist in Sydney. Her 'recipe' is from a presentation she gave to a U3A discussion group.
12 Grant, M. (2001). *Myths of the Greeks and Romans*, Phoenix, London.

Index

absentmindedness, 6, 32–40
abstract concepts, 13
accuracy of memory, 86
acetylcholine, 120, 158
actions, remembering, 12
addictive substances, 144, 159
additives in food, 142
addresses, keeping track of, 48
advertisements, 15, 16
ageing
    biased attitudes towards, 94–95
    brain cells, 103–104
    chronological versus biological, 104–5
    differences between age groups, 93–100
    how people change, 97–98
    memory lapses, 7
    normal, 80–105
    perceptions of, 95
    retirement, 98–99
    studies and tests, 95–97
    Third and Fourth Ages, 94
    variability, 100–5
alcohol, 146
all-or-nothing thinking, 65
alphabet for remembering names, 44–45
alphabetical order for organisation, 56
alternative remedies, 140–41, 143
aluminium, 118
Alzheimer's Association, 121–22
Alzheimer's disease, 106–25
    at-risk population, 109–10
    brain imaging techniques, 117–20
    compared with normal changes, 110–15

    definition, 107
    diagnosing, 107–8, 115
    getting help, 115–22
    medications, 120–21
    myths about, 108–9
    reading list, 125
    research into, 122–24
    support and counselling for, 121–22
amino acids, 154, 155
amygdala, 165, 166–67
amyloid plaques, 107, 123
anaesthesia, 146–47
anecdotes, 61–64
antidepressants, 147
anti-inflammatory drugs, 124
antioxidants, 124, 137–38, 139–40, 156
appliances and new technology, 69–71
arousal, 18
asides, 63
associations, 19–20
    see also mnemonics
    Alzheimer's, 111
    conditioning, 15
    oratory, 75
    recall, 24
    semantic memory, 12–13
attitude
    biased, 94
    positive, 105, 132–33
attitudes towards older people, 94–95
automatic actions, 3, 36–37
axons, 153, 156

balance, 103
Baltimore Longitudinal Study, 97
behaviour, inappropriate, 114–15

belongings, keeping track of, 37
beta carotene, 137
bias towards older people, 94–95
biological age versus chronological age, 104–5
blanking out, 63
blockage, 44, 45
blood-brain barrier, 121, 154
blood flow to the brain, 128, 129
blood pressure, 124
blood sugar, 135
BMI, 144
body control, 113–14
Body Mass Index, 144
Bonnet, Charles, 102
Booth, Angela, 162
brain, 151–72
    ageing, 103–5
    capacity, 152
    cells, 103–4, 153–54, 156–59 see also neurons
    effects of disuse, 98
    health, 128–29
    hemispheres, 161–62
    imaging techniques, 117–20
    lobes, 41, 163–64
    memory location, 160–68
    overview, 8
    people with Alzheimer's, 107
    physical characteristics, 152–56
    regeneration research, 168–71
    sight, 101
    smell perception, 102
brain stem, 152–53
breathing exercise, 132
bridge (game), 77
Broca's area (brain), 165
Brodaty, Henry, 122
Burns, David, 65, 66
Buschke, Herman, 115

Buzan, Tony, 60
buzz words, 70

calories, 135
car, keeping track of, 39–40
carbohydrates, 135
cardiovascular disease, 124, 135, 145
cardiovascular system, 128
carotenoids, 142
CAT scans, 118–20
categorisation and concepts, 167–68
cell birth, 168–71
cerebellum, 152–53, 167
cerebral cortex, 153, 163
characterising ingredients, 142
Charles Bonnet syndrome, 102
checklists, 37
chess, 77
Chinese medicine, 141
cholesterol, 124, 134, 142, 144
chromosomes, 123, 154–56
chronic stress, 148
chronological age versus biological age, 104–5
cigarettes, 145–46
circadian rhythm, 130
'cockpit drill', 37
cognition, 82, 156–57
'cognitive distortions', 65
cognitive therapy, 65–66, 147
cognitive training, 84–85
competitions, memory, 77–78
complex carbohydrates, 135
computerised axial tomography (CAT) scans, 118
computers, 70
concentration, 53
concept maps, 59–60, 70
conceptualisation, 12, 167–68
conditioning, 14, 15–16

conscious memory, 11–13, 28, 178
control of circumstances, 99
conversations, 41–42
Coombes, Jeff, 139
coordination, 167
coping skills, 3
corpus callosum, 153, 161
cortex, 153, 163
counselling for Alzheimer's, 121–22
counting belongings as strategy, 37
Creasey, Helen, 122
creativity, patterns in life, 103
cross-sectional studies, 96
crosswords, 109
cued recall, 86
cues
    event-based, 49
    gist of events, 84
    lack of with age, 87–88
    long-ago memories, 90–91
    recall, 24–27
    self-initiated, 87
    setting up, 48
    strategies for ageing, 86

DAT *see* Alzheimer's disease
deafness, 101
de Bono, Edward, 45
dementia
    see also Alzheimer's disease
    alternative therapies, 141
    definition, 106–7
    equated with old age, 7, 81
    getting help, 115
    incidence and prevalence, 109–110
dendrites, 153
depression, 147
detail of long-ago events, 91
development, life-long, 81
diabetes, 135
diaries, 47–48

diet *see* nutrition
dietary supplements, 138–44
    see also vitamins
    alternative remedies, 140–41
    antioxidants, 139–40
    gingko biloba, 140–41
    government regulations, 143
    medicated foods, 142
    Memory Survey, 8
    precautions, 142–43
distractions by irrelevant thoughts, 90
disturbed sleep, 130–32
DNA, 155
dopamine, 121, 158
dreams, 130
drinking
    of alcohol, 146
    of fluids before exercising, 129
drugs of addiction, 144, 159

emotional maturity, 84
emotions
    Alzheimer's and, 113
    brain structure, 166–67
    controlling, 66–67
    depression, 147
    encoding, 18–19
    importance to memories, 26
    stability with age, 99
    traumatic memories, 68
    unpleasant memories, 64
    unwanted memories, 66–68
encoding, 18–20
    automatic actions, 37
    faces, 35
    glitches in, 32–40
    memory lapses, 28
    overview, 17
    unpleasant memories, 64
enzymes, 154
episodic memory, 11–12

ageing, 89
Alzheimer's, 107
brain function, 165–66
memory lapses, 28
recall, 24
equilibrium and balance, 103
event-based future memory, 48–49
everyday activities, coping with, 114–15
exams, study for, 42
exercise, 109, 128–29, 135–36, 170
expectation of life, 94
explicit (conscious) memories, 11–13, 28, 178
eyesight, 101–2

faces, 35–36
family ties, 93
fats, 134
fear, brain function and, 166
feelings see emotions
filing and organisation, 55, 56
films, remembering, 42
finding things, 38–40, 55
fingertip management, 55
first person remembering, 66
flavonoids, 138
flight or fight response, 166
fMRI scans, 118–20
food groups, 134
food pyramid, 135–36
Food Standards Australia and New Zealand, 143
forgetting
    see also memory loss
    absentmindedness, 6
    future intentions, 5–6
    memories from long ago, 22
    'memory lapse' definition, 5
    names, 1–2, 4–5
    normal, 29, 80–105
    over time, 40–43
    reasons for, 27–29, 91
    survey, 2–3
    types of, 5
    words, 4–5
Fourth Age, 94
free radicals, 137–38
free recall, 86
Freud, Sigmund, 16
frontal cortices, 165–66
frontal lobes, 41, 163
fruit, 135, 136, 139–40
'functional foods', 142
future intentions, 5–6, 46–50, 88

GABA, 146
GBE (gingko biloba extract), 141
general practitioners, 115–116, 121
genes, 94, 123–24, 154–56
geriatricians, 116
gerontology research, 95–98
gingko biloba, 140–41
glaucoma, 102
glial cells, 153–54
glucose, 135
glutamate, 158
glycoproteins, 154
grammar and Broca's area, 165
G.R.A.S. approval, 143
Gruetzner, Howard, 121

habits, maintaining, 50
hallucinations, 102
Hampl, Patricia, 92
'hardy survivor' effect, 94
HDL cholesterol, 134
health, 127–50
    Body Mass Index, 144
    cardiovascular disease, 145

damaging substances, 145–46
depression, 147
exercise, 128–29
nutrition *see* nutrition
risks and hazards, 144–49
sleep, 129–32
social life and, 132–33
stress, 148–49
hearing, 101
heart attacks, 145
heart disease, 134, 135, 145
Heart Foundation, 143
hemispheres of the brain, 161–62
herbal remedies, 140–41
hiding places, remembering, 43
high blood pressure, 144
hippocampus, 19, 108, 130, 165
hospitals for geriatric teams, 121
how to do things, remembering, 14
humour
    and stress, 50
    and telling jokes, 61–62

ideas, holding on to, 41–43
identification numbers, 72
identity, 84, 92–93
illogical thought, 65
imaging *see* visual imaging
immune system and stress, 148–49
implicit memory, 87, 167, *see also*
non-conscious memory
inactivity, 144
individualised memories, 92
individuality, 84, 92
indulgence foods, 135
inference and semantic memory, 13
information source, remembering, 89
intentions, remembering, 5–6,
46–50, 88
interruptions to story-telling, 63

InTouch (magazine), 122
isolation, social, 132

jargon of technology, 70
jokes, 61–64

Kandel, Eric, 91, 141
keys, keeping track of, 37–38
knowledge, general, 83
Kramer, Arthur, 128

labels for food, 143
language
    Alzheimer's and, 112
    brain function, 161, 165
    semantic memory, 12
LDL cholesterol, 134
learning
    Alzheimer's and, 111
    improving with age, 84–85
    new physical skills, 90
    new technology, 69–71
    procedural memory, 14
    semantic memory, 12
lifestyle and memory, 8
limbic system, 19, 64
linking
    of new knowledge, 18
    as network, 83
list making, 47, 50, 88
locations, linking ideas to, 74–75
loneliness, 132
long-ago events
    forgetting, 22
    remembering, 84, 90–93
long-term storage, 21–22
longitudinal studies, 96–97
losing oneself, 114
Luria, Aleksandr, 76

macular degeneration, 102
magnetic resonance imaging scans, 118–20
magnetoencephalography (MEG) scans, 120
manuals, 70
maths, 112
maturity, emotional, 84
meals, 133
meaning and understanding, 18
meat, 136
medical records, 47
medications
    for Alzheimer's, 120–21
    in foods, 142
    government regulations, 143–44
    remembering to take, 49
    sleeping pills, 131
MEG scans, 120
melatonin, 130–31
memory
    ability differences in ageing, 82-90, 93, 99
    accessibility, 22
    ageing, 7
    aids, 46–50
    anaesthesia and, 146–47
    aspects that endure with age, 82–87
    aspects that worsen with age, 82–83, 87–90
    brain function, 156–57
    changes through adulthood, 97–98
    competitions, 77–78
    conscious, 11–13, 28, 178
    differences between age groups, 93–100
    emotional content, 26, 166–67
    encoding see encoding
    episodic see episodic memory
    exceptional, 74–78
    gist of, 84, 91

health effect see health
implicit, 87, 167
improving see memory improvement
individualised, 92
lapses see forgetting
lifestyle effect, 8
location in the brain, 160–68
long-ago events, 84, 90–93
loss see memory loss
myths about, 108–9
non-conscious, 13–16, 29, 178
phases of, 17–27
preserving see storage
recalling see recall
semantic see semantic memory
sleep and, 129–32
social situations, 60–63
strategies for, 31–79, 84–85
studies and tests, 95–98
synapses, 157
traumatic, 68–69
types of, 11–16
unwanted, 64–69
memory improvement, 52–79
    four steps to, 53
    Memory Survey, 6–7
    new technology, 69–71
    numbers, 71–73
    organising skills see organisation
    in social situations, 60–63
memory loss
    see also dementia; forgetting
    ageing, 81
    depression as cause, 147
'Memory Survey', 2–9
mental retracing, 38–39, 43
mental state test, 116–17
'method of loci', 74–75
microfiche, 175–76
milestones, 81

mind, 177–78
'mind maps', 59
Mini-Mental State Test, 116–17
mnemonics, 32–36, 73, 74–76
monounsaturated fats, 134
mood, 113, 147
Morawetz, David, 131
motivation, 53
movement and body control, 113–14
moving house, 57–59
multiple encoding, 18, 34
multiple tasks, 49–50
music and the brain, 161
myelin, 154
myths about memory, 108–9

names
    brain function, 165
    forgetting, 1–2, 4–5
    importance, 4–5
    from long ago, 43
    remembering, 32–36, 43–46, 60–61
neuroblasts, 168
neurofibrillary tangles, 107–8
neurogenesis, 168–71
neuroimaging, 117–20
neurologists, 116
neurons
    definition, 153
    loss during ageing, 165
    memory, 156
    networks, 159–60
    regeneration, 168–71
    synapses, 156–57
neurophysicians, 116
neuropsychiatrists, 116
neuropsychologists, 116
neuroscientists, 116
neurotransmitters, 120–21, 147, 154, 157–59
nicotine, 145

non-conscious memory, 13–16, 29, 178
noradrenaline, 159
normality, 81–90
notebooks, 47–48
numberplates, 73
numbers
    Alzheimer's and, 112
    remembering, 71–73, 75–76
'nutriceuticals', 142
nutrition, 133–44
    antioxidants, 124, 137–38, 139–40, 156
    importance of healthy eating, 134–36
    supplements, 138–44
    vitamins, 137
nuts, 135

Ohio Longitudinal Study of Aging and Retirement, 133
oils, 135
omega-3 fatty acids, 134
orators, 74–75
organisation, 54–60
    Alzheimer's and, 111
    of conflicting ideas, 57
    improving memory, 53
    principles, 54
    types of system, 55–57
overgeneralisation, 65
overweight, 144

parietal lobes, 163
Parkinson's disease, 121
patterns, numbers as, 74
pausing and reflection, 45
Pavlov, Ivan, 15
peg method of remembering numbers, 75–76
people, knowledge about, 83
peptides, 154

Perls, Tom, 94
personality, 84, 92
perspective and past experience, 92
PET scans, 118–20
phone numbers, 48, 71–72, 73
physical skills, new, 90
phytochemicals, 137, 138
pictures, turning numbers into, 75–76
PINs, 72
place, memory of, 40
planning, 54
plaques (blood vessels), 145
plaques (brain), 107–8
polyphenols, 138
positive attitudes, 132–33
positron emission tomography (PET) scans, 118–19
practise, 53
prefrontal cortices, 163
prejudice towards older people, 94–95
pressure of time, 89
priming
    with age, 87
    brain function, 167
    definition, 14
    non-conscious memory, 14–15
    role of, 29
priority list, 50
procedural memory, 14, 86, 90
prompts see cues
proteins
    diet, 135
    role in the brain, 154
Prozac, 147
putting things away, 55

Rs, three ('Record, Revise and Recall'), 42
rapid eye movement (REM) sleep, 130

rational centre of brain, 64
re-living events, 66
recall, 24–27
    with age, 86
    glitches in, 43–44
    individuals, 92
    memory lapses, 28
    multiple encoding, 34
    overview, 17
recognition, 86
reconstructions, 26–27
recording, 42, 47, 88
red meat, 136
refined carbohydrates, 135
reflexes, 86
rehearsing, 61, 62
reliving events, 61, 68
relocation, 57–59
remembering see recall
reminders see cues
research
    into ageing, 95–98
    into Alzheimer's, 122–24
    into brain regeneration, 168–71
    into cognitive training, 84
respite care, 121
retirement, 98–99
retracing see mental retracing
retrieval cues see cues
Robbins, Anthony, 15, 67–68

Sacks, Oliver, 4
saturated fats, 134
Savige, Gayle, 134
Schacter, Daniel, 18, 27, 45, 68–69, 86
Schanks, Roger, 69
'script', 67
scrutinising memory, 45, 86
self, 84, 92–93, 177–78

self-perceptions, 133
semantic memory, 12–13
    ageing, 83
    brain function, 164–65
    memory lapses, 28
    test, 117
'senior's moments', 63
senses
    ageing, 100–103
    overcoming absentmindedness, 32
    synesthesia, 76–78
serotonin, 147, 158
Shereshevski, 76
short-term memory see working
memory
sight, 101–2
sign language, 161
Silly Sentences test, 116–17
skills
    already learned, 86
    learning new, 14
    new physical, 90
sleep, 129–32
sleep disturbances, 130–32
sleeping pills, alternatives to, 131
slow wave (frontal cortex), 63
'smart foods', 142
smell, 102–3
smoking, 144, 145–46
social abilities, 112–13
social life, 132–33
social situations, 60–63
spectacles, keeping track of, 37–38
speeches and senior's moments, 63
Squire, Larry, 91, 141
stalling techniques, 45
Stampfer, Meir, 135
starch, 135
stem cells, 168, 169

stereotype of ageing, 94–95
storage, 20–23
    capacity, 23
    glitches in, 40–43
    memory lapses, 28
    overview, 17
    role of dreams, 130
stories, 61–64
strategies
    absentmindedness, 32–40
    forgetting over time, 40–43
    future events, 46–50
    glitches in recall, 43–44
    overview, 31–32
    teaching of, 85
stress, 50, 148–49
strokes, 145
studies see research
substance abuse, 145–46
supplements, dietary see dietary
supplements
'Survey on Memory', 2–9
synapses, 156–57
synchronisation, 165
synesthesia, 76–77

tacrine, 120
talks, 63
taste, 102–103
technology, new, 69–71
temperament, 3
temporal lobes, 163
temporary storage, 21–22
tests
    for Alzheimer's, 116–117
    differences between age groups,
    95–97
Therapeutic Goods Association, 143
therapists for traumatic memories, 69

thinking (cognition), 82, 156–57
Third Age, 94
third person remembering, 66
thought patterns and unwanted
memories, 65
time-based future memory, 48–49
time constraints, 85, 89
time-management, 54
tip-of-tongue (T.O.T), 43–44, 87
touch, 103
traumatic memories, 68–69
triggers see cues

'ugly sisters' as wrong words, 44
unconscious (non-conscious) memory,
13–16, 29, 178
understanding and encoding, 18
University of the Third Age (U3A), 2,
181
unpleasant memories, 64
unsaturated fats, 134
unwanted memories, 64–69

vaccine research against Alzheimer's,
123
vascular dementia, 110
vasodilators, 120
vegetables, 135, 136, 139–40
vegetarian diets, 136
video player, 69
vision, 101–102
visual imaging
    future intentions, 49
    mental retracing, 39
    names, 33
visual lobes, 163

vitamins, 137, 139–40
vitamin A, 137, 138, 140, 142
vitamin B, 137
vitamin C, 138, 139, 140
vitamin D, 137
vitamin E, 137, 138, 139, 140
vitamin K, 137

Wahlqvist, Mark, 134
walking, 128–29
weight, excessive, 144
Wernicke's area (brain), 165
Willett, Walter, 135
words
    Alzheimer's and, 112
    brain function, 165
    forgetting, 4–5
    learning, 12
    new technology, 70
    wrong, 44, 89–90
work ethic, 99
working memory
    ageing, 88–89
    concept map, 60
    failure, 5
    storage, 21
World Wide Web, 176
worry, 80–81
written aids, 42, 47–48, 60, 88
wrong words, 89–90
Wurtman, Richard, 131

Yates, Francis, 75

Zarit, Steve, 84–85